MY LIFE REWIRED

MY LIFE REWIRED

Healing Childhood Traumas and
Finding Purpose Post-Traumatic Brain Injury

ROBERT BAUGH

To request permission, contact the publisher at:
publisher@innerpeacepress.com

ISBN: 978-1-958150-77-1
My Life Rewired: Healing Childhood Traumas and Finding Purpose Post-Traumatic Brain Injury
First publication: December 2024

Cover art by Marvin C. Valenzuela, aka Davinzky Art

Published by **Inner Peace Press**
Eau Claire, Wisconsin, USA
www.innerpeacepress.com

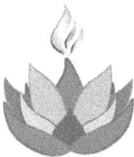

DEDICATION

I want to express my deepest gratitude and dedicate my book to my lovely wife Sheila. She has been my rock, my inspiration, my caregiver, and the very reason for my existence. Without her, I would be lost in this vast world. Sheila, you have been my biggest cheerleader, standing by my side during my triumphs and comforting me through the darkest moments of my life. I cannot fathom a single day without you in my life.

I would also like to extend my dedication to two incredible individuals, Gina Wheatly, LCSW, and Katie Berghausen, PMHNP-BC. They have been instrumental in helping me navigate the numerous traumas I have faced and have shown me that there are brighter days ahead. Their unwavering support and encouragement have been invaluable.

Lastly, I want to express my gratitude to Jill Ligon Davis, MS, CCC/SLP, CBIS, my speech therapist. It was her encouragement that gave me the confidence to start a podcast. Without her gentle push and unwavering belief in me, I would never have been able to touch and impact the countless lives that I have. Thank you, Jill, for believing in me and giving me the opportunity to share my story.

To Sheila, Gina, Katie, and Jill, this book is dedicated to you. Your love, support, and belief in me have shaped me into the person I am today. I am forever grateful for the impact you have had on my life.

TABLE OF CONTENTS

FOREWORD
BY RICK LEACH

I've known Rob for a long time. In fact, it seems difficult to recall a time during which I didn't know him! He was best friends with my brother. Both of them weren't much younger than me. They were together frequently, which meant I saw Rob on a regular basis while growing up.

I'm glad to have enjoyed my own friendship with Rob and his wife, Sheila. I believe I met her when my wife and I were out and about and ran into the two of them. If my memory is correct, it was the night of their first date. The introductions were pleasant, as expected. I'm nearly certain we walked away from that chance encounter believing they were a good fit. In September of 1998, I had the honor of standing nearby as they exchanged vows and became husband and wife. In all the years since, I've only become more convinced that God knew what He was doing when he brought the two of them together.

An ancient Greek philosopher once said, "Change is the only constant." It's hard to argue with that. Every person encounters a series of changes – they can be related to growth, maturity, or the choices we make. At times, it's simply the unpredictable nature of life which leads us down a new path. Some changes occur gradually. Others can take place suddenly. Those can be tricky to navigate. We encounter an unexpected patch of ice on a winter road leaving us with a tight grip on the steering wheel and hoping for the best.

In the pages that follow, Rob shares details about a series of life-changing events. They make up his story. You've already made the decision to check it out. I believe that's a choice you won't regret.

Despite a world which looks very different to him today, some of Rob's strongest characteristics remain as evident to me now as they did when he was younger. He is authentic. I've always considered him to be genuine, honest in his dealings with others, and never one to hide behind a facade. His written words presented here will only affirm that truth.

Rob has always been kind and helpful, willing to lend a hand to anyone in need. It's that heart for people which has led to his desire to share these life experiences with others. This might be a resource which is a blessing to you because you've faced similar trials. Or maybe you'll want to pass it along to someone you know who has endured challenges like Rob. It can be a tremendous blessing to realize you're not alone.

If nothing else, perhaps Rob's courage and willingness to share intimate details about the hardships he has faced will inspire you. It can remind you that good can come about from every difficult situation. We might develop a stronger faith as we spend more time praying and seeking strength from above. The relationships with loved ones can be enhanced as we lean upon them for support. Hindsight can provide us with clarity as we recognize growth which has taken place. Finally, there can be purpose in sharing what we've been through so that others may benefit. You might have your own story to be told!

While growing up, I was sometimes disappointed to reach the end of a television program only to see the words, "To be continued..." on the screen. I found myself anxious for a conclusion. I was invested in the story, the characters, and the outcome. As I reached the end of this book, I was reminded that there are chapters yet to be written. However, there's no disappointment in not knowing where things go from here. I'm excited to see things unfold in the future and who will be helped along the way.

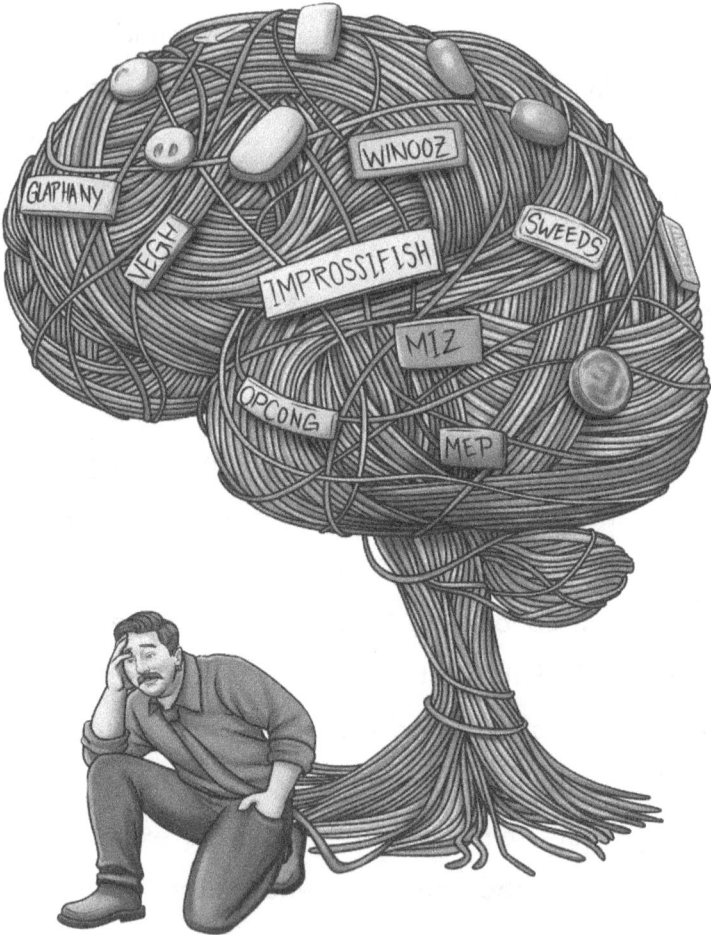

PREFACE

On July 21, 2020, during the height of Covid, my life changed forever. I sustained a traumatic brain injury at the worst possible time. It took years to discover who I was and learn to live comfortably in my own skin again. I decided to write about my brain injury and how I learned to cope with this new way of life. As I began to prepare to write, I reflected on just how many traumas I have survived in my nearly 50 years on this earth. I was blown away at how far I have come, so I decided to write about the many traumas that lead up to and include my brain injury. Many things no one in my life knew about until I shared them in this book. The reason I decided to be open and transparent about all I have been through is that I hope whoever needs to hear this message will receive understanding that you can heal from those wounds. Life is a precious gift, and we can learn to love and give ourselves grace – no matter when we become brave enough to start.

INTRODUCTION

Trauma is a deeply distressing or disturbing experience that can have a profound physical and emotional impact on a person. It can be caused by a single event, such as a car accident or a natural disaster, or by repeated exposure to a stressful or traumatic situation, such as child abuse or domestic violence.

Finding purpose after trauma is crucial for healing and personal growth. It allows individuals to transform their pain into something meaningful and impactful, offering them a sense of direction and hope. By focusing on helping others or pursuing passions, survivors can rebuild their lives and contribute positively to their communities.

As I began writing this book to tell my story of my traumatic brain injury, different traumas that happened in my life kept popping into my head. As I wrestled back and forth about sharing these traumatic events I wasn't sure I wanted to expose myself in such a vulnerable way. The more thought I gave, the more I realized that if I want to help others, I have to be transparent. This book is about how I received my brain injury, how I turned the "why me" into "how can I use this to help others," and, most importantly, how I found more than just healing after a brain injury – how I found purpose.

I will share with you how a bump in my road became a Podcast that highlights amazing people.

As you read this book, I ask that you understand that my book has been written in many layers. I compare it to peeling back an onion. Each layer will contain subjects that many of us face within the course of our lifetime. While one chapter may not fit into your circumstances, another one might. I encourage you to understand that the takeaway from the book is not one man airing his grievances to the world, but rather that you consider that every story, though filled with trauma, will have a purpose. I will leave some things open to interpretation as to how this may or may not fit into your life. I put a lot of thought to give the reader of this book a glimpse into the daily struggles that a brain injury survivor goes through. My hope is that if you are someone with a brain injury, you will see similarities to the struggles that you go through; if you are a caregiver, you will understand and read with compassion and knowledge first hand how much a survivor goes through; and if you know nothing at all, other than what you have seen on TV or the movies, that you will find that it's not what you think it is. Brain injuries do not go away in 30 minutes. My hope is what you thought of a brain injury will be totally transformed by the time you finish reading this book. Thank you for taking the time to understand and being willing to keep an open mind.

THE REWIRING BEGINS

Before I dive into how I got my brain injury, I'd like to share the backstory that ties together the reason the accident occurred at all. Ten years ago I called my wife to let her know I was going outside to cut the grass. I'd always been warned to be careful and watch my surroundings. That day I went through the same routine I always did: I began cutting the yard with the push mower to get close to the fence line before I got out the riding mower. I was outside long enough to make one pass down the fence line and, as I was coming back, I felt a sharp pain. I pulled up my pant leg and there was a wasp attached to me. I quickly flicked him off and immediately became very light headed and I felt sweat rolling down my back and felt sick to my stomach. I left the mower where it was and I went back inside the house. I called my wife, Sheila, to tell her I was done cutting grass and I really needed to lay down. I am beyond grateful that she doesn't let anything go without follow up questions. "Rob, something's not right. There is no way you can cut the grass in five minutes." I told her about the wasp that had just stung me and how I was feeling really ill and needed to lay down. She told me that was not a wise thing to do and I needed to get to Walgreens right now to be checked out. Somehow I made it to Walgreens and from that point I don't remember anything else. Later my wife told me she had a feeling she needed to get to Walgreens and asked her boss to leave early. When she arrived she heard someone saying they needed to call an ambulance because he was in no condition to drive. As Sheila rounded the corner, she saw that they were talking about me. She announced she was my wife and that she would take me to the emergency room (ER). I don't remember anything that happened in the ER, but later they advised I needed to follow up with an allergist and would need to carry an Epipen with me going forward. That may seem like a weird connection to a brain injury, but this is where it all comes into play.

I work for a company that gives me the flexibility to work from home. It is perfect for me since I work best with little to no distractions. For some people that would get old fast. But for me, a certified germaphobe who thrives on being a homebody, this worked out perfectly – it is the best of both worlds. I can still talk to my coworkers, but I am also far away from the general public. Being a germaphobe can be laughable to some people, but who else was better prepared for the pandemic than me? My wife said that very phrase to me when Covid hit.

The day that changed my life forever happened on July 21, 2020, five years after the wasp incident. It was a day like any other day. We were still trying to make adjustments to living the new norm in the Covid world. My wife had just lost her job of nearly 25 years because the company she worked with decided to close the doors. It didn't close due to Covid; they closed for other reasons. For the first time since she left high school, my wife found herself home with no job. It was a steep learning curve for her trying to get out in the field and applying for jobs that three thousand other people were applying for as well. She tried her best to keep herself busy to avoid going insane from boredom. She took walks with one of her former coworkers and did things around the house that needed to be done. She never slept till the crack of noon. She is a go-getter and is not one to waste time, so she made sure every day was packed with something to do. Not only were we adjusting to living a life of mask mandates and social distancing, we were also adjusting to her being home all day and me getting used to having someone else making noise while I work. I do remember it was a beautiful day and it wasn't extremely hot either. It was just a nice day to be alive. I made it through the day just living my best life. 2PM came and as I always do at that time of the day, I went out back to feed the fish in my koi pond. As soon as the back door opened, they all came rushing to the top waiting to be fed. I swear they know what time of the day it is. I did my normal routine: gave them their food and called them lazy hungry hounds as I always do, then made my way back inside to finish the last 15 minutes of my shift. It was smooth sailing from here. Only I didn't make it back in to finish my shift. As I began opening the back door to go inside, a bee flew by my head at the exact moment I was opening the door. And since my last run-in with a bee left me with PTSD, I go into panic mode whenever I see one. So naturally I had a knee jerk reaction and I ducked when that bee flew by my head. I was still opening the door as I ducked, and I ended up knocking myself out with the door. I don't know how long I was out, but I remember everything went gray.

When I was coming to, my hand was on my head firmly where I had just been hit with the back door. For a few moments I just left it there. I remember saying out loud, as if someone could hear me, "this is going to leave a bump tomorrow." I took my hand away from my head and my hand was covered in blood. I looked around me and blood was everywhere on the patio. It looked like I was standing in the middle of a horrific crime scene. I didn't want to rush into the house dripping with blood. Isn't it funny how in a time of crisis we still think in our OCD ways. The next best option was to get my wife's attention.

I walked over to the kitchen window, where my wife was in the process of cutting a pineapple, and I started waving to get her attention. She later told me that she thought I had wanted her to come outside to see something funny the fish were doing. When my wife came outside, she never expected to see our back patio covered in blood and me clutching my head. She asked me what had happened and all I could do was to point at the back door and kept repeating bee, head, bee, head. At first, she thought I had gotten stung by a bee, but logic quickly kicked in that a bee sting would not have produced the scene she was witnessing. Somehow, she managed to calm me down enough to find out what happened. I told her I was feeling lightheaded, and she managed to get me to sit down at the picnic table. She told me to stay put, she was going to get some towels and blankets to put down in the SUV, and get me to a hospital. The hospital was not my main concern at that moment. I asked her to get my cell phone so I could call my supervisor to let her know what was going on. She quickly ran in the house and grabbed my cell phone and brought it to me. I called my supervisor and at that point I was really having issues getting my words out. My wife took over the conversation and explained what had just happened. Without hesitation she told my wife to not worry about work and get me medical treatment right away. With that my wife went into overdrive and got me in the vehicle. I told her I felt like I was going to be sick, so she grabbed a trash can, and we began our journey to the ER.

I remember praying on the way to the ER. I kept thinking, *well this is it, this is how I leave this world.* I saw all that blood and my head hurt like someone had beat my skull in with a baseball bat. I knew there was no way this would end with me living to talk about it. I prayed for God to watch over Sheila. I asked him to give her strength to get over my death. I also asked him to find her a good man who wouldn't leave her high and dry to spend the rest of her life alone. I made my peace, and I was prepared for whatever happened next. I vaguely remember pulling up to the front doors and my wife running in to get someone to come help me get out of the SUV. I was so weak I could not walk. Before I knew it a lady came out with a wheelchair to get me. I think my wife and her both helped me out, but that part is fuzzy. I also remember the lady smelled nice. I don't know if I said it out loud or not, but I said, "Wow, you smell good." Here I am, facing uncertainty, and I am focused on how nice this person smelled. That was the last memory I had at that moment. I don't know if they registered me or shot me right back to a room. The next thing I remember is a nurse sitting next to me, explaining what she was about to do to me. They were going to numb my skull so they could put staples in the three-inch laceration to my skull. She said a lot of words but the only words that registered to me were: this is going to burn.

She administered the first shot and it felt like someone had scraped the pits of hell and threw it inside my head. I had a death grip on the rails of the bed and how I didn't rip them off the bed is beyond me. She gave me a few minutes to allow the shot to do its thing. I was relieved that part was over and hopeful that the staples she was about to put in my head would be pain free. Staple one went in and I felt my soul leave my body and smack me on the back of the head. I couldn't believe how bad it hurt. The nurse didn't want me to feel any more pain, so she decided she needed to give me another shot. My logic was since she already gave me one, this one shouldn't hurt nearly as bad since it was partially numb already. That quickly proved to be wrong. The second shot was just as painful as the first one. I had high hopes that this would do the trick this time. She gave me a few more minutes for the shot to kick in. Now it was time for the second staple. It hurt like hell; I just wanted to get this over with already. The nurse grabbed the needle again and I told her to just do the rest of the staples without the shot. She tried to talk me into letting her give me another shot and I told her I couldn't take another one. They hurt worse than the staples, so I would prefer that she do what she must do and just get it over with. Reluctantly she finished the job and laid the bed back down for me to rest. I was in and out of it for the remainder of the ER visit. I fell asleep a few times and every time I woke up my mind was racing a million miles an hour. At one point I felt someone tap my leg and ask me how I was doing. I replied that I have had better days. It was Sheila's good friend who worked at the hospital. She had come by to check in on us before she left for the day. That was the last memory I have of that day. I know we got home eventually, and Sheila got me into bed to rest up. I really didn't want to go to sleep, I was afraid that I would not wake up. I didn't want to leave Sheila all alone in this world, though I knew in my mind she would be better off without me. I didn't know what the rest of my life was going to look like. I felt tremendous guilt. She didn't deserve to have to take care of me, not yet anyway. I was only in my mid-40s. This wasn't fair to her if I somehow couldn't return to work or be a functional human being. Giving yourself grace in times like these is easier said than done.

I don't really remember leaving the hospital that day or the ride home. I only remember at some point getting into bed with a tremendous headache. My head had never hurt that badly in my life. I've had headaches and even migraines, but this was like no other pain I had ever had. In the days following the accident I anticipated that the pain would get better each day, only it didn't. Weeks went by and the headache was still going strong. As for the writing of this book, it has now been four years since my accident and the headache has been with me since that day. The biggest fear I had from day one was that I would not be able to do any other job. My ability to remember things I did even an hour earlier was impossible. My memory was so bad that at times I would cook breakfast and an hour later I would ask my wife what she wanted to eat. It is very scary to navigate through life not knowing conversations you had or even going hours without eating because you forgot to eat. Having a faulty short-term memory means you rely heavily on people around you. As for my job, I was able to remember how to do my job because I had done it for nearly 12 years. It was etched into my long-term memory, and I had no issue with that. Only my short-term memory had been affected by the incident. Shortly after my brain injury we got the news that the job I knew how to do was going away. I would have to learn something similar, but it wasn't my familiar expertise. My coworkers promised me they would have my back. They have all chipped in at some point to help me understand what I am supposed to do. Somehow, even with me having to reach out for so much help, I have been able to exceed our department standards for what I am to finish daily. My coworkers were so much help and are still there for me to this day. I've had to ask the same questions over and over, but they have always met me with patience and kindness. They have cared for me as much as my family members have.

Those first few months were rough, and I've never shared this with anyone until now, but there were many days that I laid in my bed thinking of the easiest and least painful way to kill myself. I dared not tell anyone for fear of being committed. But the struggle was real. I do not condone suicide at all, but I understand now how people get to the end of their rope and suicide seems the better option than living through the pain. Anyone who gets to that dark place of hopelessness has to choose to either live or die. Those are the two options you are left with. For me my religious beliefs are what kept me grounded just enough to not go through with ending my life. The next step was the how. How do I keep myself grounded? Like it or not, the more you are facing constant pain, the more giving up becomes a viable option. Though I never told my wife about my struggles with suicide, I desperately needed help to get through. I was nearing the point to tell her that I wanted to see a counselor, when fate made that decision for me. We went to a follow up visit with my neurologist and he suggested to us that I consult a psychiatrist and to begin cognitive therapy again (I will go into more detail later about neurology). The timing couldn't have been more perfect. Sheila began searching for a psychiatrist and just by chance one of her coworkers had a recommendation for one. We went through the intake process and that question they all ask popped up: Are you suicidal? At the moment I wasn't, I had already made up my mind that wasn't the option I wanted to take, so I answered no to that question. Once I was able to talk with her my life started getting better. It sure didn't cure my headaches, but she gave me medications to help ease my anxiety, which also helped me get more sleep. She also gave me very useful suggestions to help me stay grounded and to help me stay in a good frame of mind. For example, when I become overwhelmed, I learned to close my eyes and do deep breathing and begin to think about all of the positive things in my life, all the things I have to live for. Things like my faith in God, my wife, my friends. Anything that brings happiness into your life, that's what you need to focus on during these tough times. Another coping skill is talk therapy. It seems too simple to work, but I assure you that getting things out helps you clear your mind. It helps you to keep the positive things in your head. If your mind is filled with positivity and joy, there is no room for anything else to invade and grow like a virus. So my next step was to find a counselor who had a specialty in brain injuries. It is so important to find someone with a specialty in the area of your need. You can pick any counselor in your area to talk your problems through. However, it will benefit you more if you find someone who has experience in your specific need. They will have more resources and techniques that can be tailored specifically for you! Once I found a counselor that fit my criteria, I saw even brighter days ahead. She was able to get to the root of the things that really eat away at me. We did a type of therapy that helped me retrain my brain to replace those PTSD things of my past and helped me get out of the flight or fight that I was stuck in. I can not stress enough how important it is for you to seek help when you have problems in your life. Whether it is a brain injury, a break up, or grieving the death of a loved one. Counseling is key to recovery. One way that I find helps me when life is getting me down is to listen to music I love. Whatever type of music speaks to your soul, that brings you joy, is what I suggest you listen to. Joy and sorrow can not coexist, it is impossible. If you are a person who doesn't like music as much as I do, watch a good comedy or listen to a stand up comedian. There is something to be said about laughter being good for the soul. It is more profound than it sounds. Even the Bible says in Proverbs 17:22 that a joyful heart is good medicine, but a broken spirit dries up the bones. It is true, a merry heart really does a spirit, soul, and body good like medicine.

I don't have those feelings any longer. Counseling and seeing a therapist regularly have been helpful in keeping those options out of my head. I had to learn early on how to live with my pain. People often ask me: "How do you do it?" My answer is always the same. It is not easy. You learn how to fake a smile. Some days are better than others but the real struggle I have is when the barometric pressure falls or if it rains. If either of those things happen, I feel like my migraine has a migraine. On those days it's very hard to fake a smile.

The other issue I have daily struggles with is anxiety. Before my brain injury I was the most laid-back person you would have ever come across. Nothing bothered or upset me. I now deal with audio sensory issues that I never had prior to the brain injury. There are times I will look at Sheila and ask her if a sound is bothering her. Often she cannot even hear it. We try to time our grocery shopping to either the early morning hours or later in the evenings, so stores are not so crowded. The crowds raise my anxiety to the point where I feel like crawling out of my skin. I have had to learn so many coping skills since my injury. When I open a door to enter or leave a room, without thinking I reach the other hand out to protect myself. I am not the same person I was before I had my brain injury. The person I knew is no longer.

Some days I see a small glimpse of the person I was. Those are bittersweet days, because it makes me happy to see even a fraction of my old self. But it also reminds me how much I miss that person. This may sound totally morbid, but when you go through what I have gone through, it is as if you attend your own funeral. You literally see your old life pass away. The real work starts when you finally stop mourning the person you lost and start finding out who this new person is. In some ways I am a better person, but, in some ways, I can be downright awful. I don't intend to be a mean person at all, but I have no filter. What comes out of my mouth I have zero control over. Sometimes I hear what I say, and I am horrified by what just came through my lips. Most times it's just what I feel and believe to be true. If you want my opinion on anything and don't like someone being brutally honest, then please don't ever ask me, because you will get the full unfiltered truth. I mean no ill will by what I say. I only speak from my heart. Sometimes that gets me in trouble, but for the most part people who know me understand that I am not attacking them.

Brain injuries have a weird way of not only taking abilities from you, but sometimes you gain abilities that you didn't have before. I mentioned my love of music and playing the piano. I have played the piano by ear since I was four years old. If I liked the song, I could mentally arrange the keys I needed to press to make those sounds in my head. I would work it out from beginning to end and, once I had it, I could go to the piano and just play it. Playing by ear has advantages and disadvantages. If you want to play in a group and you only know how to play in one key then you are limited by the songs you can play. I learned to play in the key of B flat by ear. I had not played for several months after my injury. I decided that I had given up on many things I loved to do because of my brain injury, so I made the effort to sit down and play a few of my favorite songs. To my surprise when I began to play in the same key I always played in, I transitioned into a whole new key that I had never been able to play in my life. I couldn't believe what I was hearing and seeing. How did I know how to do this? It was beyond explanation. Then I decided to try another key that I didn't know how to play. I made the effort to play in the key of C. I started banging on those keys as if I had played that way all my life. And then I began playing in the key of D. Literally any song that I have ever been able to play in one and only key, I could now play in three new keys. This was an astonishing little gem I discovered after brain injury. I have always been one to look for the silver lining in every situation. Perhaps it is from all the traumas I have had in my life, but I have always been one to not stay down in the dirt too long. Some pity parties are ok every now and then, but I never wear my welcome out. My life has taught me that there must be good in every bad situation.

Writing about the issues I had with memory loss has been a bit of a challenge. For most of this chapter I had to depend solely on notes that I have taken, journal entries that I have written, and the help of my wife Sheila. For a while I kept a journal. It wasn't a daily event, sometimes it was weeks between entries. The reason I had to keep a journal was to help me remember what had been happening. My short-term memory was affected by the head injury. As I mentioned, some days I would forget that I'd already fixed breakfast. One time on my way to a dentist's appointment, before I got there I couldn't remember where it was I was going. I knew I had somewhere to be, or I wouldn't be driving, but I could not remember. I had to pull the car over and look through the calendar on my phone to see if I had something scheduled and sure enough found my dentist appointment details. Talk about full on panic mode. In the beginning of the brain injury I had a real struggle communicating with people at work. I work from home and we talk with each other through Skype or Microsoft Teams. I would attempt to ask questions and all they would see was gibberish on their end. I knew what I wanted to say but typing was a huge challenge. To slow down and type a simple sentence would take me several minutes to complete. I am sure my coworkers cringed when they saw my name pop up. Eventually my ability to type coherently improved with time; what didn't improve was my stutter. Since it took me so long to type, I would try to text using dictation on my phone. That was good in theory, but whatever you say is what gets typed. Many people received texts from me verbatim of how I said it. So you can imagine how hard it was to read something like: I I I I AM UH UH UH

ON MY WA WWWAY WAY. My stutter has since improved, though comes out strong when I am tired, nervous, or get around a big group of people. This could not be my way of life and my wife was definitely not going to sit on the sidelines and watch me deteriorate. She began looking for a neurologist immediately.

Finding a neurologist was a task for sure. My wife did her homework and tried to find the best neurologist for me. There didn't seem to be a lot of choices in our area, but she did find one who seemed like he would be able to help me. Remember this was at the height of Covid and no one could go with me to my appointment. The night before my wife drove me to the office in hopes I would remember how to drive myself the next day. That was good in theory, but by the next day I forgot the directions. I left earlier than I needed to, just in case I got myself lost. Once I got downtown, I missed my exit and kept driving. Before I knew it, I had driven all the way to a job I used to work at 20 years ago – 25 minutes out of my way. Once I realized that I wasn't going to work and I had a doctor's appointment, I turned myself around and eventually found the doctor's office. I arrived with only five minutes to spare before my appointment. I do recall meeting this doctor. He told me how wonderful he was, and that he was the best neurologist in this area. He thought very highly of himself I thought. But if he can help me, I can look past his arrogance. He took me to his office and sat me down and began asking me questions. I can't tell you everything he asked me, but even with my bad memory I can clearly tell you the first question after he asked me my name. He asked me my date of birth. My mind tried hard to remember when it was. I was coming up with nothing at all. I just could not remember. I told him I don't remember, and he looked up from his paper, slammed his pen down on his desk, and said with a very loud and stern voice, "The questions are just going to get harder from here." I felt a tear forming in my eye and I fought it with everything within me. I was not going to let this guy see me cry because I couldn't remember my birthday. I don't remember anything else he said after that. The remainder of the meeting I was on co-pilot, I just wanted to leave and bury my head in the sand. When I finally left his office, I was so upset and confused. I couldn't even remember where I had parked. I was sure it wasn't on the first level of the parking garage. I took the elevator to the second floor and I literally walked up each floor pressing the button on my key fob until I finally found my car.

I got home and my wife asked how the meeting went, I told her it was good. I wasn't going to say well he had me in tears because I am an idiot. After all, she had spent a lot of time researching so I felt this was probably in my best interest. She had lots of questions that I did not know the answers to. Even if I had paid attention, I wouldn't have remembered anyway. He started me off on a medication they give to epileptic patients. He claimed they had great success with it in removing all of my brain injury symptoms. That was not the case for me. It wasn't long before my wife said we must find someone else to help you. The plan of action from the world's greatest neurologist was to do nothing for two years and see if I get better. That did not go over well with my wife at all. This was just unacceptable, and she wasn't going to have it. She was floored that a neurologist wanted any brain injury patient to sit around and do nothing for two years to see if I just got better on my own.

She began the search again for another neurologist. And at that same time she also got me into cognitive therapy so I would have a shot at getting better. She finally came up with two doctors who had very great remarks on the website Healthgrades. She wanted me to make the call, it was important that I feel comfortable with whomever I wanted to be seen by. I looked both doctors up for myself and hands down it was the second choice. The first choice will be nameless, but he wore a bow tie. I found him on YouTube where he had several videos. The man knew his stuff, but he had to wear a dang bow tie. I am not a fan of bow ties at all, and am very OCD about this. I wouldn't have been able to listen to a word this doctor said at all. I would only be focused on the bow tie. So, the second choice it was. And, as it would turn out, it was the right call. This neurologist took the time to listen to my concerns and he had an awesome bedside manner. He was everything you wanted in a doctor.

The new neurologist took no hesitation in starting treatment right away. From the start he got me into a psychologist and a counselor to help me with my trauma. And he also got me into Frazier rehab for cognitive therapy. There was much concern about my memory issues. The first session they took my wife Sheila into another room to get some history of what I was dealing with. I don't know what was discussed but she did bring up concerns like me making breakfast and having no knowledge of it an hour later. While that discussion was going on I was busy taking tests and being quizzed later about what I could remember. All of this was done to get a baseline of where they needed to start treatment with me. The best thing about the program was they allowed me to continue meeting with them virtually over the next several months until I had the tools in place I needed to be the best version of myself cognitively and mentally that I could be.

The team I worked with at Frazier was wonderful and they did a fantastic job at getting me to a better place.

I began taking a lot of photographs and I would journal to help me remember things. I downloaded an app on my phone that was specifically made for journaling. It also allows you to add photographs as well, there is an endless source of apps that allow you to do such tasks. I used that as an opportunity to take random photos and then journal about where the photo was taken, what the photo represented to me at that moment, or any useful details that I could look back on at a later time to help me remember that moment. Even if I couldn't remember the day, I still had documentation that represented that moment of my life. If nothing else, I could relive that moment for the first time. The process helped me a lot, but it also was only helpful if I could remember to journal. My phone has tons of pictures that I have no memory of taking and no reason for taking them. I did a decent job at journaling my daily life, but I wish I would have taken better notes and had done this more consistently. There were many days I would find sticky notes on my computer that would read "call at 3:00." Call *who* at 3:00? I was sure when I wrote that reminder down that I would remember who I needed to call, but I never did. I have since gotten better at leaving myself more descriptive reminders.

My first day at Frazier I met with two counselors. They took me into a room with my wife and wanted her to be there with me. This affected her as well, so she needed to see what was going on and be a part of it. While they administered my testing to see where I was lacking, one counselor took Sheila into another room to have a talk with her. To this day I don't know what they talked about. It's possible she told me, but I have no memory of it. From the notes I took for that first session, I was having a struggle knowing what year or month it was. Sometimes I still struggle with this. The counselor who interviewed me told me when we sat at the table to tell her when it was 2:30 so we could stop the testing. I had forgotten, and she reminded me at the end of the session that I never stopped her at all. My short-term memory was struggling big time.

They gave me lots of great strategies to help me retain information and for longer periods of time. Sheila even told them how I would drive to an appointment or to the store and forget where I was going two minutes into my drive. The counselor came up with the idea to write on a sticky note where I was going and to place that on my steering wheel. If I forgot where I was going, all I had to do was look at the steering wheel and I had an instant reminder of where I needed to end up. They really had their work cut out for them, but I can say nothing but good things about their techniques. I have come a long way from where I began.

While I do still have memory issues to this day, they are much better than they were before. Mostly we have found that things tend to stick for two to three days before they are gone from my memory. The funny thing about a brain injury and memory issues is you don't have the luxury of deciding what information sticks and what doesn't. There are times that I can tell you something that happened earlier in the week, something as minor as buying a coffee from Starbucks, but then I couldn't tell you what I ate for breakfast this morning.

My new neurologist sat down with us and went through my charts to see what all I had tried prior to seeing him. He didn't want to reinvent the wheel, but he wanted to make sure he left no stone unturned. He did a full exam on me, something the "wonderful" doctor never did. I explained to him that since the day I hit my head I have had a headache around the clock. It was 24 hours a day, 7 days a week. He asked me how I would rate my pain, and I finally felt prepared for the first time. One thing I did from day one of my injury was to grade my headaches on a scale of 1-10. 1 being the least amount of pain and 10 being a full-on migraine. I had tons of data to provide to him and this was helpful in him deciding where to begin. The first several months I had a daily range between 4 and 6. If we had a major drop or raise in the barometric pressure or rain it went straight to a 10.

It was debilitating in the beginning, and I would be lying if I didn't say I would lay in bed some nights and wish I would just die. At one point I finally made up my mind that I needed to sink or swim. While I really wanted to sink, the love I have for my beautiful wife is what kept me going.

I want out of this pain I am in, but the thought of my wife spending the rest of her life alone forced me to say: start swimming! I eventually learned how to fake a smile. On the days that I was a 4 or a 5 it was a cake walk. But those days that I felt the marching band in my head, it was pure hell, and it took a long time to force a smile on those days. My days in the 4-6 range came to an end when I got my first Covid shot. I won't debate if they work, don't work, or if it is all a conspiracy, that is something you can decide for yourself. I can only speak of my own experience. After that first shot my daily average headache was a 7. In fact, after that first shot, it never dropped below a 7 again. Then came the second shot and booster, that was a whole new beast. My headache score went to a 10 and stayed there. Some days it dropped to a 9 but it mostly stayed at a 10. The last time my headache was an 8 was Friday April 21, 2023. I have no idea what was different that day, but that was the lowest my headaches have been since the last Covid shot.

The first course of action he wanted to try me on was medications. We tried everything FDA approved at that time, and nothing worked. After all the failed attempts with medication we moved on to botox injections. My first thought was I am going to look so young. But that wasn't what this was for. The injections go into your skull, neck, and shoulders. This didn't sound like something I was going to be excited to do every three months. The doctor explained that it typically shows results on the third go around. If I felt no relief after that, he would stop the treatment. There was no need to keep going if I didn't have any relief after that.

I made up my mind that I would not Google or look up on YouTube what the procedure consisted of. And I am glad I didn't. My wife took off work to take me to my appointment for moral support. Little did I know there would be a total of 31 injections. I felt sick to my stomach when he told me that. But, I was in it to win it. If the injections worked, I would gladly suffer through every three months. I braced for the first injection and the immediate pain shot through my skull and throughout my body. I had a death grip on the exam table and my arms were shaking. All I could do was close my eyes and try to go to my happy place. With each injection I was counting, 30 more to go, 29 more to go.

Then, out of nowhere, he turns on a fan and starts asking questions. What did you have for lunch, my wife didn't answer. I thought, *come on Sheila, answer the man because I do not feel like talking*. After six or seven injections he gave me a break to get my composure. When I opened my eyes, there stood my wife holding on to the door with all her might. She just about passed out from watching what I was going through. I wanted to laugh because I was the one in pain, but the truth of the matter is that she loves me so much she couldn't bear to see me going through so much pain. On the way to the car, she said, "Rob I love you, but next time I am staying in the waiting room." And she did!

I felt no relief at all from the first round of injections and I was hoping that maybe round two would at least give me some type of relief. The next time I was scheduled for my injections I wrote on the calendar "torture day." I wasn't looking forward to it. And, as it would turn out, the second round of injections also failed. I had zero hope of round three being any different, and it was still the same outcome. No relief in sight for me.

After giving it some time, our next course of treatment was nerve block. This was not nearly as painful as botox. The length of time you could feel relief was different for everyone. I polled people in various support groups I am a member of and got everything from no relief at all to two days, two weeks, and two months. It was just so different depending on the individual. I sadly got zero relief from the shot, and the chances of a second round of treatment being any different were pretty slim. So I opted to put that treatment to bed and move on.

The continued course of action would be to continue seeing my psychiatrist every three months and my counselor every other week. I am very satisfied with my counselor as she is very attentive and has had some great suggestions to incorporate into my life to help me deal with my anxiety and panic attacks. I haven't had nearly as many panic attacks as

I had in the beginning. That monster will probably always be a part of my life, but at least I have the tools to tame it when it rears its ugly head. We have incorporated EMDR (eye movement desensitization and reprocessing), which is a psychotherapy treatment designed to alleviate the distress associated with traumatic memories. Those are big words that meant nothing to me when I was asked to do this treatment. I had to Google and watch videos to see what it entailed. In my translation it helps people to heal from the symptoms and emotional distress that are a result of disturbing life experiences. Studies have shown that by using EMDR therapy people can experience the benefits of psychotherapy that once took years to make a difference. This therapy shows that the mind can in fact heal from psychological trauma like the body recovers from physical trauma. It's a way to retrain your brain to help you understand that those bad things can't hurt you anymore.

My first EMDR session was harder than I had anticipated. They really want to figure out your triggers and then use those triggers to bring up those emotions so the brain can be retrained to deal with it. The theory is that you can retrain those bad responses to certain situations so your brain doesn't go into fight or flight more when triggered. It's a way to tell your brain that while this is a bad situation, it is one you can handle. Something I will go into more detail on later is one thing we focused on during that first session

— my earliest memory of a traumatic event, which happened to be sexual abuse from a neighbor. This neighbor who I will never name used to play the song *Pretty Woman* all the time. That song was my trigger. If the song ever came on the radio, I would have to change the station quickly or turn it off. The emotions attached to that song hit me all over again when I heard it. It immediately makes me relive the mental and physical abuse all over again. So that was the trigger my counselor used to get me in that state of mind. We did several sessions in a row until I was able to calm the emotional roller coaster going on inside my head down to a soft roar.

My counselor encouraged me to pay close attention to my dreams, visions that popped into my head, or whatever. Keep them in mind, write them down, or whatever it takes so we can discuss it in our next session. If I am being honest with myself, I really didn't expect anything to come up at all. In my mind it happened, I lived it, and I just don't want to think about it. I really doubted I would get any visions popping into my head or any weird dreams. As it turns out, I was wrong because I had the strangest dream that night. I dreamed that I took 2-by-4s and nailed them to the toilet. I had no idea at all what this could possibly mean. Did I hate toilets for some reason? It just didn't make any sense. I talked to a coworker the next day and I told her I thought the dream was not connected to what happened to me as a child. And then the vision happened. It was like a still picture displayed in front of my eyes. It was stripes, now it's worth mentioning that I hate stripes. I hate them with a passion! People in my life won't wear stripes around me because they know how much I despise stripes. To give you context of just how much I hate stripes I will take you back a few years. When I was a teenager, my brother, older than me by seven years, who did not know at the time and still doesn't know of the sexual abuse I faced as a six year old, made a comment that our family dentist looked like a child molester. Well that seed was planted and as you can imagine I never went back to the dentist again. It would be 16 years before I had to see a dentist because of a tooth issue. It took everything in my wife to get me to agree to see a dentist. The first appointment did not come to pass. I arrived early and walked into the lobby and the entire waiting room was striped wallpaper. I turned around and went back to my car and called them to cancel my appointment. They asked if I would like to reschedule, and I told the lady that I would check my schedule when I got home and call back to reschedule. I never called back, and I have a feeling she knew she wasn't going to hear from me again. So back to my vision of stripes. I saw the stripes morph into wooden slats, and that is when the light bulb went off. The neighbor had tied me to the bottom of a set of bunk beds. He started off by doing something

I don't want to mention, but halfway through he stopped and asked me if I had to go to the bathroom. I told him I didn't need to go. I can still see the pupils of his eyes as he got into my face and said, if you pee in my mouth I will kill you, so are you sure you don't have to go? I told him maybe I should go to be safe. He escorted me to the bathroom that was across the hall, he stood at the door watching me the entire time I did my business. I took my sweet time, I was hoping that he would just say never mind, someone would interrupt, or something would happen to stop what was happening. That never happened, so I finally finished my business and went back to his room to be tied up once again. The entire time he did those things to me I just stared at the slats that supported the upper bunk and tried my best to tune out what was going on. The connection was finally made, the 2-by-4s represented those slats on the bed. My mind was trying to prevent me from using the restroom by placing those 2-by-4s on the toilet lid. It was such an eye-opening moment. All I could do was think *wow just wow.* I asked my counselor if my hate towards stripes could have been the slats on the bed, as they looked like stripes. And we both concluded that it is most likely why I have had such a distaste for stripes.

Having a breakthrough moment doesn't mean you are healed; it means you understand the whys. We are still working through childhood trauma. I can say that I am in a better place now than I was a year ago. I still have my moments though, and I suspect that maybe I will always have my moments. But perhaps they will be fewer and farther between. I know I am better equipped to handle the emotions than before. I am confident that I will never be in a dark place that I can't see any way out. There was a time in my life that I was ready to give up. During my freshman year of high school my grandmother was diagnosed with cancer. It was so hard dealing with the idea that she wasn't going to be in my life much longer. She was my rock, my everything. I never told her what happened to me as a child, but when I was around her, I felt safe. Unlike the safety I ever felt from anyone in my life, except for my wife. When my grandmother passed away, I was devastated. How could I go on? Who would protect me from the evils of this world? I had the entire summer to think about my grandmother's death. Every day felt like the day before. Would the void in my life she left ever grow smaller? I didn't think so and in fact I was sure of it. The summer was growing shorter, and I would soon start my sophomore year. That scared me to death, and I know that probably sounds crazy. But I was really scared to start a new school year.

I had made up my mind that I was not going to be going back to school and in fact I wasn't going to be going on with life. I waited for the night that my parents went bowling and my brother would be at work. I had at least two hours to end my life. I contemplated leaving a note to explain why I couldn't be a part of this world any longer. I thought long and hard about it, but I did not want my parents to know of my childhood abuse. I felt that I just needed to go with me to the grave. I could not put the pain of my death with the pain of knowing their child had to carry such a burden all his life. So with that I was ready to do what I had to do. I went to the kitchen and searched for any cleaners that I could drink that would do the job and do it fast. Back then I was a young, dumb kid and we didn't have the internet to Google anything, so I just used my best judgment. I found a gallon of bleach and I thought, yep this should do the trick. I made my way to the bathroom and locked the door. I was ready to get it over with. I sat the bleach on the bathroom sink and as I reached to unscrew the top I heard a voice say to me, "I never gave up on you, why are you giving up on me?"

You hear people all the time say they heard God speak to them. Maybe they did, maybe they didn't. I am a Christian and I do believe in God. I had never heard his voice and I am not claiming that was his voice. But I promise you I heard a voice as clear as can be say those words to me. With that, I stopped unscrewing the cap of the bleach. I can still feel the warmth of the tears that were slowly making their way down my cheeks. I sat down on the floor, and I saw what I can only describe as an angel come through that locked door. I saw no face, no wings. Only light and the shape of a body. I felt no fear at that moment. I only felt peace and comfort. Like the comfort you feel from a tight hug from a loved one. Eventually I picked myself up and returned the bleach back to its place in the kitchen, and I went and laid on my bed and just stared at the ceiling. I'm not sure how long I laid there. But I just kept thinking about the experience I just had. I felt like I could give life another chance and I would just roll with the punches as they come.

Having to relive all those childhood traumas was difficult to say the least. But you must do hard work to see results. It took 43 years for me to finally forgive myself for what I thought I let happen to me. The truth is I didn't let this happen to me. It was going to happen; I can see that now. Would it have been days, weeks, or months? Who knows, but this obviously was something my abuser had thought out. He was just waiting for the right time to put his plan into action. My only regret is carrying this burden for so long. If I could go back in time and talk to my six-year-old self I would have reported the incident immediately. But you can't live your life in the past and play the what if game. I played that game all my life and one thing I have learned is no matter how many times you play that game, the result is always going to be the same. The only thing you gain from playing what if is putting yourself through constant torture over and over again. The only thing I can do at this point is forgive myself for allowing someone to have control over my life. That is one thing that I will never allow to happen again. And that is probably why I have trust issues. It takes me a long time to be open to people. Once you crack that shell I have around me, you have a friend for life.

Someone recently asked me what advice I would give to someone who is just starting out on their brain injury journey. I told them to get into a support group. It's the best thing I have ever done, and I wish I hadn't waited so long to join one. It was two years after my brain injury before I finally got on Facebook and found a support group to join. My advice is to join more than one group. There are many groups out there and I have found that not all groups are created equally. There are some toxic groups and if you are looking for support you do not want to put yourself into a group of people who will drag you down. The purpose of joining a support group is to connect with others who are going through what you are going through. You need a support system to have people lift you up when you are down and vice versa. Yes, you will also need someone to listen to you when you need to rant about the frustrations of a brain injury, or whatever it is you are facing. You must find the right balance. I found that in some groups you can post a question and never get a response. While others you can ask and within seconds you have 20 people offering up advice and their personal experiences. It's funny to say this, but I have more friends now than I did prior to my brain injury. I have a great network of friends all around the world who will lend me their ear in a moment's notice. If you are lucky enough to have an in-person support group to attend, I would highly recommend it. I was trying forever to find one near where I live and there didn't seem to be any. I was going through my second round of cognitive therapy – my first therapist had warned us that down the road I would probably need more therapy again. I guess it is kind of like a car… every now and then you might need to get it in the shop for a tune up. My lovely wife happened to find a brochure of a new group that was just starting up. My prior therapist from Frazier rehab had moved to another state and it wasn't going to be possible to see her anymore. The new group that had just formed was two ladies who used to work at Frazier rehab, and they had decided to branch out on their own. From the start I already felt comfortable knowing they came from Frazier.

My second counselor was fantastic. She was super patient with me. I know I can be a handful, so she had her work cut out for herself. For once I took pretty good notes, partially because my wife was with me, and she was my cheerleader. She would say, "I think you need to write that down." And, as always, she was correct. I often ask her if she ever gets tired of being right all the time. One thing my wife brought up with my therapist was she has to remind me of people who have passed away. There were instances when I would come home from town and tell her I saw someone who had passed away. Then she would have to tell me that the person was no longer living. This may seem morbid to some, but we came up with a death book. I wrote down the names of people in my family who were no longer alive and the date they passed. It was something that I would review from time to time. I still struggle with this to this day. The other issue my wife told the therapist was everything happened yesterday. At least that is what I would say. I went to the movies yesterday, when in fact it was two weeks ago. For some reason, anything I can retain in my brain becomes something that had happened the day before. That is an ongoing struggle that we battle about and probably will for a lifetime. This is how a brain injury looks, it's different for everyone. We might share the same injury, but it can manifest in so many ways. I like to think of a brain injury as a snowflake, because no two are alike. When we were near completion in my sessions, my counselor told me another one of her patients wanted to start up a support group for people with a brain injury who still work a job. It took me two seconds to say, "I'm in!"

I was a little nervous about meeting new people, but I wanted that connection. I'd never been in a real support group before, so I didn't know what to expect. It was very laid back and I discovered that the others had the same concerns and frustrations that I had.

In one session I was complaining that I laid in bed every night trying to find videos on YouTube of survivors having a conversation about things brain injury related. I would find tons of videos of doctors saying this is a brain injury and these are the symptoms. I didn't want to hear from a professional who had never had a brain injury tell me what it was like to have one. I was living it; I already knew what it was like. The thing I was looking for I just couldn't find. When I stopped complaining, the counselor in our group looked at me and said, "Well, if you can't find it then you do it." I said, "Who me? I don't even know how to upload a video to YouTube." But then I said, "You know what, yes, I will do it." I went home that night and I looked up a video on YouTube to find out how to upload a video to YouTube. This was the start of the podcast "Life Rewired" which I will talk about in detail later.

As I end this long chapter, which I hope gives you a good overview of what I've been through, I would like to ask you to reflect on your own life. What got you to where you are? My bet is that most people in my shoes would – in a millisecond – reverse what they'd gone through if given the chance. Not me. That's not because being injured is a good thing, it is because what I learned about life, and myself, through the process has been invaluable. I learned that when life knocks you down, that's when you find out what you are made of. Am I a person who is going to sit back and let the punches keep coming my way? Or, do I get up, put the boxing gloves on, and say, "Ok let's do this!"? There is work to be done and I am in it to win it. I still put my gloves on daily, and I still fight that fight. One day I may even get to retire those gloves. And you can too! Never give up the fight, be open to receiving help from your friends and loved ones. And know that on those days that you are too tired to put those boxing gloves on, it's ok to tag someone in.

MAN PLANS AND GOD LAUGHS

As the old saying goes: Man plans, and God laughs. I have heard that saying so many times in my life. I used to think it was such a rude statement to make. I thought it was a slap in God's face. The more I think about this, the more I am convinced that I had taken it all wrong. What does this saying mean to me? We have a vision of how things should be in a "perfect world." We make plans and expect them to go exactly as we plan them to go. Where the God laughs part comes in is that we are not living in a perfect world. From the beginning of man we often fail to see our plans through exactly as we want them to go. Along our journey we are often thrown so many curve balls that many people abandon their plans and totally give up what it was they were aiming for.

My life was going perfectly well when I was forced to make a 180-degree turn four years ago when I knocked into that door. The life I had known was never going to be the same again. When tragedy strikes it makes you totally reevaluate the things that matter the most, and you quickly learn to not sweat the small stuff. Things like how perfect the lines in your yard are when you cut the grass. Those things no longer matter. Now you are just thankful to get the grass cut.

Trauma can leave you so bitter inside and it makes you just so angry when you see others around you enjoying their life to the fullest. It can also make you appreciate the things that you are still able to do; you understand that things are bad, but they could always be worse. I have joined many support groups since my brain injury. I have seen all walks of life. People who must have help to get dressed. People who are bound to a wheelchair. People who have lost the ability to work altogether. Some people can bounce back right away. Some people seem to keep facing setbacks. I quickly learned that brain injuries come in all shapes and sizes. They cannot fit into a perfect little box.

A week before I suffered my brain injury, a coworker who I really respected told me about a position that was about to be posted. She was on my team for a few years and we had become good friends because of a project that was forced upon us. Our company had been doing something wrong and it cost the company a lot of money in fines. They chose the best employees they trusted to complete the project. We alone were the only ones who could work on this project. It was very tedious and time consuming, so we were not held to a production metric because of the sensitivity of the project. The bottom line was it had to be done right, or the reality was we would end up losing this business.

After the project was completed my friend posted out to another department. Every time an opening came available she tried her best to recruit me, but I remained faithful to the team I was on, and quite frankly change really scared me. The longer I thought about it I kept leaning more towards posting out to that position. It really was something totally different and it was something I knew I could do. When she asked me again to apply, I finally said yes. It just so happened that she had the ability to put in a very good word for me. She had quickly moved up the ladder of success and her recommendation held a lot of weight. Chances were the job was mine for the taking if I wanted it. And I really did want the position. I had such an awesome supervisor – the best that you could ever ask for. Someone who cares about their employees. It was such a hard decision, but I was determined that I needed to advance my career.

The position was posted about two weeks after I had my brain injury, and by that time I couldn't write a complete sentence to save my life. My speech was not any better either. I didn't have *any* business applying for a job at that point. My memory was so bad and there was no way I would even be able to learn a new job had I wanted to. That left me bitter for a long time. I never thought I would get through that anger stage, but I did. I was really upset that I let myself get excited for a new position and then it all changed in the blink of an eye.

In the beginning, just after the injury, my family was understanding. They called daily or sent my wife Sheila a text to see how I was doing. Members of the church we belonged to sent cards filled with words of encouragement. But, as the days went by, the calls stopped coming. The texts eventually stopped dinging as did the beautiful, handwritten cards. Everyone had made up their minds that enough time had passed and I had to be better by now. Little did they know brain injuries don't work that way. It's not like falling and scraping your knee. Those heal after a few days and eventually the scab falls off and, if you are lucky, you won't have a scar to remind you that you need to be more careful and maybe stop doing stupid things.

The truth is that with brain injuries time doesn't heal all wounds. And it has been proven that with time even more symptoms can pop up out of nowhere. For the first year of my injury, I was able to say numbers properly. One day I woke up and I could say one through nine just fine. But after nine, everything came out one-zero, one-one, one-two, and so on. Even for me to say 12:13 it will come out "one-two, one-three." The doctors who I have seen agree that it is connected to a condition called aphasia. Aphasia is a language disorder that affects your ability to speak and understand what others say. You might have trouble reading or writing. It usually happens suddenly after a stroke or traumatic brain injury.

Not only do I have issues with numbers, but I also have problems with getting the right words to use for common items. For example I know what a Q-Tip is, but my brain does not allow me to find the word Q-Tip in my vocabulary. So instead of saying Q-Tip, I will compensate by describing the item rather than saying the word for it. In my house I will ask my wife where the ear sticks are. She has been around me long enough that she knows exactly what I am asking for. This would pose a real problem with people who are not around me very much. They would probably look at me like I have lost my mind. This is just a small glimpse into how the brain injury has changed my life.

The big takeaway I found in having a brain injury, and several other survivors have echoed this feeling many times, was: the people in your most inner circle, and that can be family, friends, or coworkers, are the ones who seem to have less compassion for you than a complete stranger would. I have found that strangers ask me more questions about brain injuries than some of my family have ever asked me.

Brain injuries are no respecter of race, religion, creed, or color. And unlike a broken arm or leg it cannot be seen other than the symptoms they leave behind. Such as short term memory loss, fatigue, headaches, confusion, loss of balance, sleep disorders, mood swings, sensory issues, blurred vision, anxiety, the list goes on and on. Where the big trouble lies with brain injuries is lack of education. Most people go their whole life without ever having or being around someone who has a brain injury. Their only education on a brain injury is seeing someone hit their head on a sitcom, they forget who they are, and in 30 minutes they hit their head again and now they are healed. How I wish that were the case.

I wanted this book to be all about my brain injury and all the baggage that comes with it. The more I wrote, the more memories of past traumas kept spilling into my mind. I had no clue about all the traumas I had been through in my life. The more I write and take notes, the more memories flood into my head. For that reason, I decided to start from the very beginning to give you a glimpse into what real trauma looks like. I will not try to wrap this in a pretty little bow and pretend that many parts of my life were not, to be blunt, abuse. I wanted to be as open as I possibly could. I know that the things I have survived, and many others have survived as well, are things most people do not talk about, especially men. I hope after reading this book, if you have lived through similar circumstances, that you will consider doing the work to heal those past pains. We can't erase our past, but we can heal and grow.

My story isn't finished yet and my brain injury doesn't define who I am. I may have a different way of doing things than I did before. I have learning issues that I may never overcome. But that will never define me. I am a positive person trying to make a difference in the world. I am a firm believer that I want to leave the world a better place than I found it. My story is so much more than just my brain injury. In many ways my brain injury saved me from myself. I was a ticking time bomb and had no clue how much anger and rage I had pinned up inside me. I hope that in being transparent with my life I will help others grow in theirs.

To put everything into perspective as to how I have healed, I am writing about traumas I went through that many people have either had firsthand experience in or at least knowledge of someone who has gone through such things. My story is about my brain injury, but also about healing. Healing has been a common thread throughout my life. It will also be a common thread throughout this book. Trauma is something that we all face at some point in our lives. Very few people make it from birth to death without picking up some kind of baggage that must be dealt with. I encourage you to keep an open mind and know that there is always a light at the end of the tunnel. As the old saying goes, it is always the darkest before dawn. I want everyone who has faced those dark times to know that there is an explosion of light waiting for you just around the corner. My brain injury may have been a bump in the road, but I have learned that even roads covered with potholes can be filled in. Something beautiful can come from the least likely of places. Keeping a positive mindset has gotten me to this point in my life. The easiest thing to do is nothing. Nothing is an easy approach and requires zero effort at all. But remember that something will never come from nothing. If you want victory, you must be willing to fight. There is no battle you cannot win if you keep pressing on. You will see during the various battles in my life that there were many times I could have easily thrown up my hands and called quits. Some people wouldn't have blamed me one bit. But I am a warrior, a traumatic brain injury warrior! Quitting is not an option for me, and I hope it isn't for you either.

You may not hear many people who have survived a traumatic brain injury say this. But in so many ways, this injury changed my life for the better, even though I deal with pain every waking second of my life. It has given me so much to offer to the world. It has helped me to change people's lives. There are many great things on the horizon that would have never been possible without my brain injury. Things that I never dreamed would be possible. And it all started changing the moment I found my purpose.

LIFE REWIRED, FINDING PURPOSE FOR THE PAIN

YouTube helped me learn how to make videos, but the beginning of my Podcast journey was a little rough. My first video was just myself telling my story of how I got my brain injury. After that I put up a few videos of songs I had sung and me playing the piano. I was still trying to find my footing. I knew what I wanted to do was to have other survivors join me. I wanted to have them tell their story. I needed a place where people could use my platform to be heard. And I wanted my channel to be educational for survivors who are just discovering their new life with a brain injury and to educate non-injured people. I remember before I had my injury, the only thing I knew about traumatic brain injury (TBI) was what I saw depicted on TV and in the movies. And guess what? It is nothing like what you see on TV. There are a few movies that get dang close, but in real life you can't just switch back and forth by bumping your head again. It is nothing like that. Some people get back to normal or as close to normal as possible, while others have a lifetime of recovery. One woman I met, a lady in her 40s, told me she had a book on her nightstand she created that had in big bold letters on the cover the phrase "You are not 12 anymore." That was her daily reminder. If she woke up and saw that, she would remember that she had a TBI and she knew what the day looked like for herself. If she didn't see it, she would get out of bed and get ready for school. Because, in her mind, she thought she was 12. She needed that reminder every single day to get her on the right track.

The Podcast allowed me to start asking people in my online support groups if they wanted to come on and tell their story. I had a few people take interest, but nothing was ever concrete. I was determined I was not going to give up. I kept making videos and I was at 10 subscribers for what seemed to be an eternity. I figured I must be doing something wrong, and decided I need a second set of eyes. I posed the question in my group and asked if anyone would be willing to look at my channel and give me their honest opinion of it. A very nice lady named Ashley reached out to me and said if I sent her the link she would look at it. She watched a few videos and told me I was too all over the board. She told me I needed to be consistent with my videos, and she was right. There were too many areas I was covering. I had my personal story which was great, videos of me singing, and other random videos. I could see why my YouTube channel was confusing to people. They didn't know what my channel was about. I thought it was great advice and I thanked her for taking the time to look at it. Then I asked her if she would like to be a guest and tell her story and she said yes. I didn't have a program I used to record the internet with, so she suggested we use Zoom. We had a plan in motion, and I was ready to roll.

Ashley and I hit it off from the first time we met. We just had such chemistry together. We had something unique. My wife knew me before I had my brain injury, her husband didn't know her before she had hers. We each had something we could bring to the table with different perspectives on the subject.

Once we finished recording, I asked her if she would like to be my co-host. I really wasn't looking for a co-host as I had planned to do this all on my own, but I felt like we could really move some mountains as a team. She said yes, and I am so thankful she did. Ashley is excellent at being brutally honest. If she thinks something is a bad idea, she will tell me in a heartbeat. I respect her for that, because I want to make sure what we are doing will reach both brain injury survivors as well as educate people who don't even have a clue what a brain injury is. I find that most people who have never been around someone with an injury have very limited knowledge of what it entails. It isn't what you see on TV and in movies. You can't totally be mad at people who are insensitive to brain injury survivors. You don't know what you don't know.

To make our podcast successful we didn't want it to be two people who just showed up and only threw out facts on what a brain injury is. That's something that anyone can go and look at. We wanted to make it something that was in a forum of presenting facts, but how can we brainstorm and have solutions to common issues we all face. We also wanted it to be a platform for other survivors to present their survivor stories. That was a great way to show other survivors that even though our lives are not what they once were, there is still hope and healing after a brain injury. Our third and most important goal is to be educational to the rest of the community that doesn't know the real struggles of brain injury.

Ashley has been such a driving force behind the podcast. She is so much better at doing research and has better communication skills than I do. She comes up with really great ideas and we both make it a team effort to figure out how to best present the information to our audience.

Coming up with a name for our new show was a clever mistake. I think we both had ideas and neither of us was 100 percent sold on the title. I told my coworkers and asked them if they had any suggestions for names. I think I got a few good ideas, but nothing really said this is it. I told them I wanted it to be something brain injury related. Something that would express what I felt. I feel like my whole life has been rewired. I wasn't the person I once was. I joked that maybe I should call it Life Rewired. Everyone loved it. Hands down they all said Life Rewired should be the name of the podcast. A name was born, and we went full speed ahead.

I am so thankful for Ashley's input in the show. To this day she still uses the phrase "this is your show," but I always correct her that this is our show. It may have been my idea, but she takes her role in the podcast seriously. She wants to make sure that what we do is professional, educational, and entertaining. And she never fails to deliver in that department. I have been able to book great guests to come on the podcast. That is one of my strong points. Ashley asks me all the time how I was able to get certain guests. I just tell her that I am persistent. And I never leave a stone unturned. There is no one I will not reach out to.

The podcast hasn't just helped us to help others. It also began a new friendship that I would never have had without it. Ashley and I have become like brother and sister. We text all the time and keep each other updated on what's going on in our personal lives. We are both each other's support person and it's wonderful. It's such a great feeling to know that when you do something that you beat yourself up over you have a person you can reach out to and share in your disappointment and tell you it's ok. If you are reading this book and you have a brain injury and don't have your go-to person, please find that person. I can promise you that if you are in any kind of support group you will find someone willing to be your person if you just ask.

I don't expect to be some famous YouTuber who can quit his job and do this as a full-time thing. I am not doing this for fame or fortune. I am doing this to spread awareness of brain injuries, TBIs, and CTE (Chronic Traumatic Encephalopathy is a neurodegenerative disease associated with repeated head injuries, particularly in contact sports and military service) – anything that is brain injury related. Most people will never have to deal with living with a brain injury, but chances are at some point in your life, a friend, coworker, or loved one will have some form of a brain injury. Education is key and knowing how to treat (or help) someone with a brain injury is important. You can't support someone with a disability unless you know something about the disability. Sure you can help with day-to-day things, but you need to know things such as anxiety triggers, and the plethora of other symptoms one might have.

Life Rewired is still growing, and we are still finding our audience. There have been a few times that I wanted to throw in the towel. I would ask myself: *Am I making a difference?* And out of the blue I would get a nice note from someone who happened to find our podcast. The outpouring of positive feedback that we have received has put more fire into me to keep going. One email I got was from a lady who had been a survivor for 14 years. She found one of our podcasts we did on what not to say to a brain injury survivor. She showed it to her husband. She went on to tell me that he always blames her brain injury as an excuse every time she forgets something, or the fact that she gets fatigued easily. He constantly told her that she was using her brain injury as a crutch, and he honestly didn't believe she was as bad off as she claimed she was. She told me that not only did her husband watch the podcast in its entirety, but he also came to her and told her how sorry he was for the way he discounted her symptoms over the years. He admitted that he treated her that way because he was ignorant of what all comes along with a brain injury. He failed at doing his homework. The fact that she took time to write to me to thank me for doing the podcast made me realize that it doesn't matter if I can change 10 million lives. If I change anyone's life for the better, then I know that what I am doing to raise awareness is worth all the blood, sweat, and tears I put into it.

Here are a few comments and messages that we have received since beginning the podcast. I've omitted the commenters' names to protect their privacy.

YouTube Viewer: A great example for how important educating the general public about brain injury is! I have her book and recommend it! Only through education can we understand brain injury and all other non-visible issues we humans have! Being vulnerable is very difficult for us all! Thanks for sharing and bringing insight into traumatic brain injuries!

YouTube Viewer: Wow wonderful video. All the videos on your channel are fantastic.

YouTube Viewer: I've also had a brain injury. Well done with your recoveries. My point is that you said Veronica is unable to work. I think she has difficulties with certain challenges and these difficulties may need some help from someone else to overcome. I think that is different to being unable to work. In my opinion, being 'unable to work' and 'having difficulties working' is a change in mindset. If you start with a very simple job, do it well, and improve everyday, this allows for growth in the future. If you approach a situation thinking that you have difficulties, then the best course of action is to learn how to overcome those difficulties. If you approach a situation thinking that you are 'unable to work,' then there isn't a logical next step to move forward...

YouTube Viewer: Hi Rob. I'm 15 years out of my TBI due to an auto accident. My husband, son, daughter, and I were in our Mustang when we were T-boned by a semi on the highway. I just wanted to put it out there that understanding a TBI is one thing, and I appreciate you educating others, thank you. Another element I struggled with for many years was accepting my own injury and what changes came along with it. I pushed, too hard, to just keep going. Now that I am learning so much more about it, I find myself completely grateful for your efforts!

I am forever grateful for every comment that I receive and for every email or private message. Every time I question myself: *am I making a difference? Is what I am doing even worth it?* I read those comments and it humbles me. It is a great reminder that I am not doing this for me. I am doing this to be a voice for all brain injury survivors. For stroke victims, for people with CTE, or aneurysm survivors. Everyone who has suffered a brain injury deserves the respect to be acknowledged that they are still a human being, someone who has feelings. We may not be who we used to be, but we are still somebody and our injuries should not be discounted.

Who knows where this next chapter of my life will take me. I am doing something that is therapeutic for me, and I am helping others to share their stories. I've talked with authors, counselors, people from England, Newfoundland, Australia, just all walks of life. And we all have that one commonality: brain injury. We understand what each other is going through. We know compassion and patience. That doesn't mean we are good at practicing patience, but we know about it. My hope is that the podcast can go on for years, and with the power of the internet, this is something that will still be here long after I am gone. I pray that even after I am gone, people will still be able to find some nuggets in the words I leave behind – something to inspire them to be their best self, something that will inspire them to do a random act of kindness for someone else in need. Whatever it is that a person needs to get out of my messages, I hope that they receive it. As I said before, it is my passion to spread awareness. I am sure I don't always hit the mark. But I like to think that I do more often than not. I pray that I am doing a good job at communicating what needs to be said.

I must admit that in the beginning of my brain injury life, I had just a few friends. My fear after the incident was that I would never have anything in common with another person again. Through the podcast I have made so many great friendships. A few people I have had on the podcast I don't hear from anymore, but just about all the rest I have been able to build friendships with. I have more friends now than I did before my brain injury. The podcast has not only been therapeutic for me, but it's given me so much more. That is why I am always thinking about what I can do next. How can I make the podcast better? How can I make this better for all survivors? I am constantly trying to check off all the boxes. Will I ever meet the need of every situation? Probably not every single one, but I do feel that I can help the masses. What I started as a way to show people how my life changed as a brain injury survivor has become my own personal field of dreams.

I didn't want the podcast to be the only platform for survivors. Somehow it seemed like a great start, but I felt there was more that I could be doing for survivors. Having been in several support groups I noticed that many of them have admins who frown on survivors sharing things like podcasts, or a book they have written – anything that would help a survivor in promoting something they were working on. That just didn't sit right with me. As a survivor I want to help anyone I can. If someone wants to sell a secret family recipe to make a few bucks I have no problem with that. I know there are many of us who cannot work any longer. So If I can help someone feel loved and accepted and even make a little money, I am all for it. So for that reason I created a support group for survivors as well. I encourage them to promote whatever it is they want to promote. The only stipulation I have in my group is to be kind to each other. Friendly debates are ok, but there is no room for hate in our group.

The phrase it takes a village took on a whole vision for me when someone commented that they wished they could watch the YouTube podcast. They were vision impaired, and they could only listen to audio. It was something that I should have figured out from day one, but as I said sometimes it takes a village. The moment I saw there was a need that wasn't being met, I had to fix that right then. I had no idea how to get the YouTube videos onto listening platforms, but I was determined that I would figure it out.

Within a week I had purchased the program I needed to make this happen and I began transferring the audio portions of the podcast into files to upload to Spotify and to Amazon music. As long as one person is listening to the podcast on either of those platforms, I will continue to keep it updated. I do not want to have one person left out. I spent too much of my life sitting on the sidelines, letting people walk all over me, and always feeling left out. For that reason I will always do whatever I can do to help others.

PODCAST STORIES

To give you an insight on just how different brain injuries are, I wanted to include a few stories from the podcasts that I have done so far. Each one is unique but you will also see similarities in the various symptoms that come along with a brain injury. With every interview I do, I always walk away with some nugget of wisdom, inspiration, and appreciation for being brave to say I am not going to sit around and do nothing. One time I had another survivor tell me that it was foolish of me to think that I could change the world. That really hit me hard and it stung. Then I started going through my emails and reading the comments that people had submitted to me and I was once again encouraged. I know I can't change the world, but I can change some. It really reminded me of a story a pastor once told us in church. There was an old man walking down the beach and he saw a little boy in the distance. With a closer inspection he saw that waves had washed up thousands of starfish. The little boy had taken it upon himself to reach down and throw the starfish back into the ocean so they could survive. The old man walked up to the little boy and said, "Little boy, how foolish of you to do such a wasteful task. There is no way you can save every one of those starfish." As the little boy reached down to pick another up, he looked at the old man and said as he threw the next one back into the ocean. "I know I can't save them all, but I made a difference for that one." That story has stuck with me some 30 years later. It still rings true to me. I know I can't make a difference for the whole world, but think of the people who I have touched. That makes every effort I put into my podcasting worth it all.

One thing I learned very early on in my new endeavors as a podcaster is to do a screening on your potential guests. In the beginning I would let anyone come on to tell their story. While I do believe that every story deserves to be told, not every story is necessarily for a broadcast type platform. Some guests are not comfortable in front of a camera and that can lead to a very awkward conversation where you are doing all the talking and having to put words in your guests mouth. As a host you want each guest to shine bright. You also need to think of the audience you are trying to attract to your program. The audience isn't tuning in to listen to how encouraging the guests' story is. The guest needs to have content relatable to why someone is listening in the first place. You also must be sensitive to the people who are viewing your content. Just because someone has a great story to share, it could be a trigger for your audience. You can't be afraid to pre-screen your guests and let them know that certain parts of their story might be more harmful to a viewer than it will do good.

One interview that we did was on a very sensitive subject, and had I done a pre-screen I would have been able to advise the guest that it was just too graphic to share with others who may have anxiety or PTSD. How this person received their injury is even too hard for me to talk about to this day. Once the interview was over, Ashley and I had a conversation, and I told her that my heart went out to our guest, but I had a hard time holding back the tears. Ashley told me that I hadn't done as great of a job as I thought I had masking my feelings. She told me that the expression on my face told it all. She even had such a hard time with it and it gave her so much anxiety to hear what this poor soul had gone through. Ashley has never watched the interview to this day. I had to sit through it a second time since I am the editor of our podcast. It was just as hard sitting through it again as it was the first time. At least during the editing process, I didn't have to hold back my emotions. I had to stop several times during editing to have a good cry.

I struggled hard all week going back and forth if I should air the video or not. For every reason I came up with to axe the whole interview, I came up with another one that was just as valid to let it air. When it was all said and done I made the decision to let the interview air and I gave it a heavy trigger warning at the beginning. I owed it to the guest who had poured their heart and soul into telling their story. I also felt that if it even helped one person, then that would make it worth it all. This was the only video I have done that I didn't care if it got good ratings or not. The only thing that I cared about was the potential to save another life.

Much to my surprise the video is the third highest rated video we have done to date. Even though my gut was telling me no, my heart was telling me I had to do this. It ended up being the right decision, but it taught me a valuable lesson to ask more questions and never be afraid to gently tell someone that their story is too deep for our audience. Just because their story isn't right for our format, it doesn't mean it still can't be told in other ways.

One of our earlier guests on the program sought us out. She was a brain injury therapist from England. My initial thoughts were that she probably wanted a free promotion. I have no problem with guests coming on my podcast to promote anything, I just was a bit confused why someone would be so kind to come on our podcast to help us out and wanting nothing in return. I guess that's just my nature to doubt people's good intentions. I am quite sure it has to do with my past traumas. I took a leap of faith, and a little cyberstalking, to see if the person was legitimate or not, and I told her I would love to have her as a guest on the podcast. Her name is Natalie Mackenzie, aka the Brain Injury Therapist. She was such a delight to have on our program. The only problem that stood in our way was we are on the east coast, and Natalie is from England. So the time we were free to do our interview with her was actually 11PM in England. But she assured us that it was not a problem. She just wanted to come on to our podcast and help spread awareness. Natalie told us how health care works in England, and it really makes you thankful for what we have here in the states. If you were to have a brain injury in England, you typically must wait upwards of two years before you can get in for treatment. Two years is a long time to wait, especially when your recovery needs to begin immediately.

I was so thankful that Natalie stayed up late to give us a wealth of knowledge that she had gained in all her years dealing with brain injury survivors. The podcast was a big hit and really spoke to the hearts of other survivors. It also gave some pretty good information to caregivers as well. Natalie taught me that I need to be a little more trusting in people's intentions. Not everyone is out for themselves. She may never know how much I needed to be proven wrong. I am not a person who has to be right in every situation. I am comfortable enough to admit when I am wrong.

Even though our podcast is meant to educate people who don't know what it's like to have a brain injury, and a platform for survivors to tell their stories, Natalie opened me up to other interviews that I would have flat out ignored, simply because I didn't take time to hear the person out because I felt their intentions were selfish or self-promoting. I would welcome her back to our podcast any time she wants to be a guest.

I couldn't write a book on brain injury awareness and not talk about the most replayed episode that we have done to date. We did a show called "What not to say to a brain injury survivor." We hadn't really touched on this topic before, and it's probably one of the most obvious subjects to talk about. In our support groups there are always comments being made like can you believe someone said this or that to me. And without fail hundreds of comments would always follow with things that were said to them. My co-host Ashley and I took a poll in a few of the support groups and asked what is something that people say to you that is insensitive but they do not realize it. We had so many replies that it was nearly impossible to read them all. We had our data available and were ready to tackle the elephant in the room. This show was totally meant to be educational to people who do not have a brain injury. The number one thing that was a common thread from all of the survivors that we polled was the comment: "But you look fine." That comment seems harmless and is most likely intended to be a compliment to a survivor, however, it is more hurtful than helpful. When you have a brain injury, that is something that is internal. You cannot see it. That is why it's called the invisible injury. When you tell someone that phrase, it's actually dismissing their injury all together. The biggest misunderstanding about brain injuries is people assume that if you look fine, then you are ok. So my advice to anyone who ever speaks to someone with a brain injury, to just speak to them as you would speak to anyone else. It's perfectly fine to ask them about their injury, trust me when I tell you that we all love to tell our story, we all need to tell our story. As an outsider the best thing you can do is listen and have compassion. Kindness goes much farther than someone who tries to tell you how you can get better from something they are not going through themself.

I was proud that Ashley and I did that podcast. It really resonated with a lot of people. I got so many private messages on Facebook, comments left on our YouTube channel, and emails. An email I received that I reread from time to time was from a lady who had suffered for over 15 years with her brain injury. Her husband is her caregiver and constantly accused her of using her injury as an excuse and surely her symptoms were never as bad as she claimed they were. She went on to tell me that she asked her husband to watch the episode on what not to say. After viewing the episode he actually apologized to his wife and thanked her for showing it to him. From that day on he never discounted her symptoms or accused her of using them as a crutch to get out of doing things she didn't want or couldn't do. That one letter spoke volumes to the work that I am trying to accomplish with the brain injury podcast. That gave me hope that what we are doing is really changing lives.

The one constant in my podcast journey has always been purpose. I don't want to do a topic or an interview just to have content to put out. I like for everything I do to be relevant so my audience can either learn something they didn't know before, or to lift their spirits to see that they are not alone in their brain injury journey. I have talked to many people who left me feeling so much better, not because I am doing better than they are, but because they either taught me something I didn't know before, or they were just simply amazing people. One recent interview I did was with a young man named Christian Licciardi. His father Joe had somehow learned about my podcast and sent me a message asking to be on the program. He sent me a video to watch of his son's journey and it had me in tears. Christian had been fighting migraine level headaches for a very long time. He had visited the ER several times and was ultimately sent home with medication and no answers. The last trip he made to the ER his father demanded that they do more intense testing to get to the root cause of the issue.

That may have saved his son's life, because they did find the root cause and it was from a sinus infection – the last thing you would ever think would cause a brain injury. It wouldn't be long after that before Christian ended up in a coma and began the fight for his life. Eventually Christian came out of the coma, but the doctors told his family that he would never be able to walk, talk, or see ever again. Christian proved the doctors wrong. He not only had a strong will, but he had a praying mom and dad who never gave up hope.

During our interview the topic of purpose came up a few times. Like I've said, I am always looking for a purpose. While we were talking I had a vision of Christian teaching other survivors how to fly fish. I said Christian who knows, maybe someday you will have your own camp and teach others how to fish. Once I said that, his mouth dropped and his father got so excited. Joe said that is his dream. He actually had a business plan before he had his brain injury to open a wilderness camp and teach people who are depressed or have a brain injury how to fish. When he said that, I got goosebumps and cold chills. I had never met this kid before. I had no knowledge of his goals or plans in life. That to me was a total God moment. If you had asked me to guess what his dream profession would be, never in a million years could I have come up with a camp for brain injury survivors.

I was so glad I did the interview that day. I never told Joe or Christian just how bad I felt. My headache was well over a migraine level, but when I make a promise to someone to do something, I keep that promise even if it means I have to suffer. I have watched the interview at least a dozen times since that day and I can't tell that I was in pain that day. Sometimes the ultimate sacrifice of oneself to help another person is worth it in my opinion. I could have easily told Joe we need to do this another day. After spending time getting to know this family I have no doubt that he would have been more than happy to reschedule. I am sure Joe would have said to me what I have always told everyone else. Be kind to yourself.

That is something that I say almost on a daily basis. And when you think about it, it makes total sense. Why do we constantly put our own happiness on the back burner? Why do we treat ourselves in a way that we would never treat others? Friendships come and go, the people you are working with today will most likely work for another company within the next 5-10 years. The one constant in your life is YOU! You are with YOU from the day you are born until the day you die. How you treat yourself is just as important as how you treat others. Joe may never realize it, but the kindness he showed me off camera reminded me that I need to be kind to myself.

Doing the podcast has taken me all over the map. You never know what state the next interview will be from. The most recent interview I did ended up being closer to home than I had ever imagined. I happened to be scrolling through one of the many support groups that I am a part of and I came across what I thought was a newspaper article headline that read, "Columbus native overcomes severe brain injury, depression to become successful attorney." I thought that was really cool because Columbus, Ohio, is not far from where I live. Up to this point I would get excited if I interviewed someone that was in the same time zone as me. His name was Cameron, and at first I wasn't even going to ask him to be on the podcast. Not because I have anything against lawyers. In my mind I never thought someone in that profession would want to speak to some guy with a small podcast. But then I started reading the comments under the article and the first comment I read made me see red. The person said congratulations but I hate attorneys, or something to that effect.

I honestly expected to see the author come back with something in his defense. And he would have had every right to say hey buddy not all attorneys are money hungry snobs. But all he did was like the comment. That really blew me away that he didn't get defensive with this person who made such a horrible blanket assumption that all attorneys are the same. That's when it struck me that while I didn't share the same view as the man who made such an insensitive comment, I had already made the assumption that Cameron wouldn't want to talk to me. I had jumped to a conclusion before I ever asked him if he would be interested.

I finally congratulated Cameron on such a great success and told him that I also have a brain injury and started a podcast and asked him if he would be interested in being a guest. It wasn't long before I got a response that he would love to be a guest on the podcast. Not only did he turn out to be the nicest person I have ever had the pleasure of speaking with, he lived even closer than I originally thought. As it turns out, the newspaper headline was actually a thumbnail to a news story that was done on him by a local television station. I clicked on the link and much to my surprise this TV station was one that is in our viewing area as well. He wasn't from Columbus, Ohio, as I thought, it was Columbus, Indiana (my home state). He had since moved within about a 10 minute drive from my house. I thought it was so cool that I have talked to people around the globe, and when I wasn't searching, I found someone in my own back yard.

Cameron had originally intended to be a minister. But one day all that changed in an instant. When he was 18 he was enjoying a day on his skateboard, something he had probably done several times in the past. And he ended up being hit by a car. This left him with a severe traumatic brain injury. He had just proposed to his now wife a month prior and everything was looking up for him before the accident. Once he came out of his coma he had to relearn so many things, including his fiancé's name. She didn't hesitate for a moment. She took her wedding vows seriously before they ever walked down the aisle. She told him that she would still marry him if she had to push him in a wheelchair the rest of his life. That right there shows you that there is still a thing called true love. Something that you don't see nearly enough nowadays. Some people never make it to the better or worse before they call it quits and run their separate ways.

Cameron decided to change gears and go to law school. He was determined that he was not going to let his injury define who he was. If I recall correctly, six months after his injury he got married and then started college. The things he has accomplished in a short period of time, some wouldn't have done in a lifetime. Now nine years later he has four children, three of whom are triplets. You know he is a man of faith when he can have a brain injury, triplets, and a stressful job all at the same time.

A few things I found so interesting about Cameron was that not only did he survive and make such an amazing recovery from the accident, he invited the person who hit him to his wedding. If that is not the best example of how to be a Christian and forgive those who have hurt you, I don't know what one is. And the other thing I found interesting was he eventually went to work for the same attorney who represented him. Cameron told me he and the attorney just made some kind of a connection from the get-go. After speaking to Cameron for a while, I could totally see how that would have happened. He is just a down to earth guy who makes you feel like the conversation you are having is the most important thing going on in his life. Speaking to him is just like speaking to an old friend you haven't seen in years, but yet you pick up right where you left off.

As if Cameron hadn't already conquered the world by now, he decided to write a book about his injury. The book is called *Saving the subject, How I Found You When I Almost Lost Me*. The book has a very unique cover. There is an image of a skull on the front cover, with part of the skull missing on the left side. The image is actually a scan of his very own skull. He had lost about a third of his skull due to the injury and had to have surgery. He obtained an image of his skull and had a 3D model of it made and proudly displays that in his office.

We scheduled a time to record the podcast and I wanted to get the book before we recorded. Cameron must have known that I wouldn't have enough time to finish the entire book before we met, so he had the foresight to email me and tell me what chapters and even down to specific pages I should read that would help me. I've never had a guest that did my research for me, but I was so thankful that he did. Before we ever met, I made sure to read the things he thought would bring the best interview possible. Once I had that down, I started from the beginning.

Cameron's writing style is so unique and none like I have ever seen before. There was just so much thought provoking statements that I connected with. There were little hidden gems along the way. His book is so deep and it covers so much more than a brain injury. Everything from fatherhood, marriage, and spiritual guidance. There is something in this book that literally anyone can benefit from.

I asked Cameron's permission to read something from his book that spoke to my heart, and he gladly said yes. He had written a letter to himself and it was a letter that covered perfectly all the emotions that I went through on my journey through my new brain injured life. I try to explain to people how it feels, how lonely it can be, how mad you get at yourself, even how mad you get at others, possibly jealousy because they live a "normal" life, or what

I perceived to be normal. Yet everything I once knew was gone. How I longed to even look in the mirror and see even a glimmer of the life I once knew.

I managed to get through the reading, but I got so emotional and had to really fight back the tears. The words I had read said perfectly what I could not say. To find the right words to describe it, was near impossible for me. It was almost like Cameron had written my life story. I was so grateful that our paths had crossed, that I had read something that just spoke to my soul. There is no doubt in my mind that our chance meeting was just a coincidence – our paths were destined to cross. I may not have the impact on his life that he had on mine, but the conversation we had I will cherish for a lifetime. It ended up being the longest interview I had ever done. And to be honest I think I could have talked to him for another three hours without blinking an eye. I can not wait to see where life takes him. I think the sky's the limit for Cameron.

As I have stated several times, I have many more friends now than I had prior to my brain injury. I have a lot of that to thank because of the podcast and the various interesting people that I have had the pleasure to interview. The first author that we had on the podcast was a lady named Dawn Corbelli. She and her daughter had been in a car accident several years back. Dawn had the foresight to journal every step of their recovery and was able to write a very wonderful book about it. If you find yourself looking for a good inspirational healing story, I highly recommend you read her book *A Miracle a Day, One Day at a Time*. After my accident I wasn't able to read books. Before the accident I used to find a good book and read it within two days. My ability to comprehend what I read was very limited, so I just gave up reading altogether. Once I booked Dawn on our program I felt I owed it to her to buy the book and attempt to read it and take tons of notes. Once I got the book in the mail it sat on my desk for three days before I ever cracked the cover. Time was nearing the interview and I thought I would read the titles of the chapters and do my best to skim it so I could at least write a few notes down as if I had taken the time to actually read it.

I read through the chapter titles and quickly decided that I was going to attempt to at least read the first chapter. My thinking was that the bulk of her story was going to be in that first chapter. If I took the time to read that, then I would have a good understanding to ask questions. Once I started reading I literally could not put the book down. I had to reread several times so I could understand, but I was actually hooked. I read all of the first chapter and I just kept on going. It took me twice as long as it normally would have, but before our interview I was able to finish the entire book. I felt so proud of myself for doing what I never thought I would be able to do again. By the time I met

Dawn for our interview I felt like I was a part of the family. Her style of writing was so inviting and made you feel like you were one of her family members that she was sharing her journey with. We have become really good friends since our interview and Dawn is the one who gave me the nudge to sit down and begin writing. During our interview I joked that I was going to write a book and she got so excited and said joyfully, "YOU SHOULD!" The words "YOU SHOULD" stuck with me that day. It took several months before I finally decided to sit down and begin writing my story. I know how lonely I felt during those first few years and that is why I finally decided it was time to be open and honest so I could help as many people as I could.

LEARNiNG ON THE JOB

Being a newlywed couple you think life is smooth sailing. I was a naive person and thought life would be a bed of roses. You work hard, make a decent income, maybe have children. I am what people have called the eternal optimist. However, there were a few more bumps in the road than I expected. Adjusting to married life was a new chapter in my life that I embraced fully. Shortly after we got married, I started a new job. It was a time in my life that changed for the better and was a much-needed distraction. Over the next few years, I changed jobs a few times, for more money and new experiences. I finally landed a job that had a lot of potential. At first it wasn't the ideal job, but eventually it became the job of my dreams. I would tell people I "GET" to go to work, instead of I "HAVE" to go to work. It wasn't the highest paying job, but I made decent money. My first position at the company was as a debt collector. I hated every second of it, but I had my eye on other positions that were not on the phones. I had spent much of my career tied to a phone and I just didn't like talking to people. If you have ever had to deal with the general public, it can be a blessing and a curse. I was great as a debt collector and my boss praised me all the time for my ability to get people to pay their debts. My calm soft voice must have played a part in that. One time a lady joked with me that I could talk Santa into delivering packages at Easter.

The company was growing fast, and our office was starting to get jobs from our California office. They wanted to move as much work to those of us out east because the average pay was cheaper in the east. The day finally came that a new position was coming, and it was for payment research. This is where a customer has sent in a check and didn't put their account number on the check and no one knew what account to apply the funds to. I know you probably think: just look the name up on the check and bingo you have your customer. It wasn't that simple. That theory was applied prior to it escalating to me. Sometimes people don't have a checking account and they ask or pay a family member or friend to send in a check. Money orders was another type of payment to research. When our location got the job and took the department over, it was just three of us doing this. We had someone from California come out for the day to train us, but there was no training manual. So, my good friend and coworker Lenoard and I took on the task of just writing a manual. We worked long, hard hours, but we finally made something of quality and anyone who knew nothing about what we did could just take over without any hiccups.

Things could not be going any better and I was such a happy camper – until the news broke that our CEO had done some shady things and put the company in a very unfortunate situation. A new CEO was brought in, and he did major housekeeping. I survived seven layoffs, and with each layoff that meant more work was piled on my desk, along with my normal responsibilities. How long could I keep doing this? I would arrive at work each day and wonder: *Is today the day? Will I be looking for a new job tomorrow?*

I kept my mouth shut at home about my fears. I never have been one to lay all my cards on my table. My wife knew work stuff was bothering me, but she couldn't get me to confess to what exactly to save her life. Eventually I started having massive headaches that went on for several days. I began to stutter, and bad. My wife was so concerned that she called my coworker Leonard and said please keep an eye on Rob. She explained to him what she noticed in me. Leonard was also seeing the same thing when I would say good mo mo mo mo morning.

Leonard watched out for me; he had my back. He was the kindest person you could have ever wanted to call your friend. Leonard had a heart of gold; I would dare you to find one person who cared as much as he did and who would defend you. You don't find many people like him nowadays who are true friends. Leonard was very concerned about my speech. I didn't know until later that Sheila had called him. Leonard cared so much about my health, that he snuck behind my back and let the manager know what was going on, which resulted in me being called into her office. I thought for sure I was being fired. I was greeted with a hello Rob, I just wanted to have a chat with you, you have done nothing wrong. She continued to tell me someone had let her know that I might be a little stressed. I replied who who who who ma ma ma me? I could not hide behind my words at this point. She saw firsthand that I was in fact stressed out. She told me she was allowing me to have a few weeks off for family medical leave to heal and rest up. So reluctantly I agreed it would be for the best.

Sheila was starting to get concerned about the headaches and the progression of my stutter. It seemed that every day my condition was getting worse. Sheila decided that she was going to get answers and got me in for testing. After we got through all the testing, it was determined that I'd had a nervous breakdown. It made sense though, after surviving as many layoffs as I did, and it didn't really shock me. It turned out that what I needed was time away from work and to get some overdue rest.

This was a very valuable lesson to have learned and something I believe can be applied to all of our lives, especially men. Men have a tendency to bottle up their emotions. We feel like we have to be strong and put a brave face on. Doing this does not change the situation. I have not once heard of any outcome changing because someone refused to talk about the situation and let all those feelings out. By bottling up your emotions you are giving yourself a false sense of emotional safety. Research has shown that bottling up your emotions causes a disruption of your sleep. It causes an increase in depression, stress, and anxiety. You get sick more often and you are more prone to headaches.

One thing that can greatly help, and I say it many times in this book, is therapy. I am not suggesting that every time you have a bad day or someone makes you mad that you have to run to counseling. Finding someone who you trust to be a listening ear is oftentimes all you need to just vent your frustrations. Many times when you need someone to listen to you, you are not seeking their invaluable words of wisdom. Sometimes you just need someone who cares enough about you to listen without judgment and give validation to your feelings. This is advice I should have taken when I was going through so many layoffs at work. I didn't have to share the burden alone. Speaking my concerns to my wife wouldn't have made her love me any less. It wouldn't have changed the outcome at all. What it would have done would be to get out all those bad emotions, allow me to sleep better, and to be less cranky about a situation I had zero control over. It would have saved a lot of money in medical bills as well. Venting to your wife is not the same as going to therapy, but the bottom line is to not keep it all inside and avoid what you are going through.

I did get rest for those few weeks I was off, and I returned to work with the attitude that I can only do whatever I can do in eight hours. If the work doesn't get completed, that is beyond my control. And I kept that attitude for several more weeks until the other shoe finally dropped. The company I had once loved to work for, but totally despised now, shut the doors for good in our location. I was relieved, but nervous for my future. The big relief was that I no longer had to worry about losing my job anymore. I finally crossed that bridge; it was like a big weight lifted off my shoulders. But now it was replaced with another weight: finding a new job.

I didn't have to wait long to find a new job. I was out of work for six weeks. Had I known at the time I would easily find a new job, I would have enjoyed my time off work a lot more. And as it turns out, the new position I accepted was also something that I really enjoyed doing. I worked at a bank in a small department preparing loan documentation. The job was great, and I enjoyed working again. The people I worked with were laid back and we all got along so well. I was relieved that I had a job that wasn't so stressful. Some days could weigh on you when you had three lenders wanting their documentation all at the same time, but for the most part it was so enjoyable and having coworkers I enjoyed being around was a bonus. The only drawback with my job was the pay. I had to take a big pay cut and it was getting harder to see myself working at this company for the rest of my life.

Eventually I had the good fortune to have someone refer me to the company where I work now. I was excited to start my new job. The big pay raise that came with it was probably 90% of the excitement. I attended a five-week training class on my new role. It was very overwhelming at first, but before training ended I really got the hang of it. Once out of training I got to my desk, and I was ready to conquer the world. Little did I know how strict this department was. They wanted the noise level to be very quiet at all times, which didn't really bother me that much. Too much noise distracts me anyway, and I do work well when it's quiet. I can live with this. Then I found out once a month you must work a 12-hour shift. Let me tell you, those days I was ready to jump out a window by the tenth hour. Now let's talk about accountability. If you were not at your desk, they provided you with lovely 8½-by-11 cardboard signs that read: break, bathroom, lunch, one-on-one, meeting. *Is this daycare?* I thought. Then the day came when my supervisor called me into the office. I thought about how I could be in trouble. I am exceeding the production goals. I have 100% quality, and last I checked I didn't call anyone any mean names. I was asked to take a seat and I thought, *Well, it was fun while it lasted. I guess I am getting a box and a pink slip today.* My supervisor proceeded to tell me that she had noticed that I had not made any friends. Um, excuse me? What do you mean by make any friends? "Well, you sit at your desk all day and you do not talk to others. You have 90 days to make a friend." She wrote this information up in a document and signed it, had me sign it, and then put it in my employee file.

As I walked out of the office I was almost in tears. Did I just get in trouble for not talking? And this from a department who warns people about talking too much? You could have knocked me over with a feather. As I sat down at my seat, the lady whose desk butted up against mine looked up at me and she said, "Is everything alright?" I just looked at her, I guess she noticed the bewildered look on my face. I replied, "Will you be my friend?" She looked at me like I had horns growing out of my head, "Um sure, is that what the meeting was all about?" I said, "It sure was. I have 90 days to make a work friend." You could have knocked her over with a feather at that point, too. She said,

"Sure, I'll be your friend." From that day on we did become good friends. We both agreed that we hated this job with everything that was within us.

As it would turn out, my supervisor did me a favor and she didn't even know it. The friendship I sparked with my coworker eventually got me out of that department from connections she had and into a role that I still am working now 16 years later. And I do love what I do now, and I love the people I work with. My team must be the greatest group of people I have ever worked with. You sometimes hear the phrase 'my coworkers are like family.' It sounds so cliché, but this is the truth. I love these people like they are my brothers and sisters. We laugh together, cry together, celebrate our wins, and lift each other up at our losses. If you are ever lucky enough to like the people that you work with, be sure to let them know from time to time how much they mean to you. You spend more time with the people you work with than you do with your own family. Having a great job is important and having a good income is just as important. I encourage you, if you have not already, be sure to build relationships with your coworkers. Community is so important, having a sense of purpose and belonging is what we all desire. And you can achieve that by simply being yourself and being there for your coworkers when they need you.

There were some real important lessons that I learned in all of the highs and lows of my career. Job security is never a guarantee, and if I allow myself to be stressed out if my job will be eliminated, it will never change the outcome no matter how much I stress or worry about it. I have learned that it is so much better for my mental health to just enjoy the journey and live each day to the fullest. Tomorrow is never promised to any of us. But how we approach any situation whether it be a job, health, or finances, the outcome is still going to be what it's going to be. That I cannot control, but what I can control is how I react and accept the situation for what it is. Should the day come that the door closes on your employment, you have experience to carry with you to your next adventure in life. The road to your future is only as bright as you let your light shine.

LET'S HEAR IT FOR THE CAREGIVERS

The importance of having a caregiver in my opinion is 50% of your recovery. It helps to have a cheerleader and someone to have your back. I have said from day one that caregivers are the unsung heroes. And I am forever grateful to have been blessed with the best caregiver.

Most people do not realize when you have a brain injury that it doesn't just impact the person with the injury. Their life's not the only one that changes. A caregiver now has to think for two people. They have to be proactive and be two steps ahead of you at all times. Being a caregiver is not a job that someone signs up for and says I can't wait to do this. It's like being a parent. It's not a part time job. There are no holidays or weekends off. It's a 24/7 job until the injured have recovered, and in some cases it is for life. I want to emphasize the fact that being a caregiver is very stressful. An interesting statistic is in cases where a spouse has suffered a traumatic brain injury, 50-75% of those marriages end in divorce in the first two years after the injury. If that doesn't tell you how stressful being a caregiver is, nothing will. I don't throw that statistic out to scare people. I bring this up so this will be something on the mind of the caregiver as well as the injured. This is the time when all bets are off and you show up and prove to the world that you took your vows seriously. I may be over optimistic, but I truly believe that if one can survive a traumatic brain injury, everything else is just an obstacle you haven't beat yet. With a big emphasis on yet. Remember that you are a team. There are two people in the marriage, not one. Every day will not be a picnic, but approaching someone with grace and compassion when you probably would rather hit them upside the head will make all the difference in the world. As much as I let the caregiver have their moment of glory, I also want to remind the person with the injury to never take that support for granted. Be thankful for that person in your life who says I am with you no matter what happens. There are a lot of us who have no one to help carry the load. So always be thankful and tell them often how much you appreciate them. Kindness works both ways.

I have had the privilege of speaking with a few caregivers in my support groups as well as the podcast. One caregiver I interviewed admitted that it was a daily struggle.

Her daughter had been born with a brain injury and it took several years for it to be diagnosed. For the most part she does an amazing job as a caregiver, and I could tell she had tons of patience. She admitted that some days are harder than others and when she fails, she is the first to admit it. And it is always welcomed with grace and forgiveness.

After that podcast aired, someone reached out to me and thanked me for giving equal time to the caregivers. She thought it was so special that someone took the time to discuss what it's like being a caregiver. I assured her that I see firsthand what my wife deals with daily. I know I can be a handful at times. But I couldn't have a podcast about brain injuries and not give the caregivers their fair dues. I told her that her husband may not say it, but I can guarantee that he is very appreciative of everything that she does for him. She had been trying to encourage him to get back to playing his guitar. I told her to never stop encouraging him. When the time is right, and he is ready, he will pick it up again. And when he had his confidence built back up, the door was always open for him to come on the podcast to let his light shine.

I do hope that the words I speak on the podcast are uplifting and encouraging to others. I hope that people share the information with others, especially with the neurotypical people who tend to discount our symptoms. Those people are my main target audience. I want to be inspirational as well as educational. What I am doing is not meant to be for entertainment for 20 minutes a week. I want this to be life changing. I want people to walk away thinking about how it would feel to be a brain injury survivor. I want the survivors to walk away feeling like they have been heard.

I asked Sheila to give her perspective or thoughts on how I have changed as a person, the things she sees me struggling with, or how she helps me navigate through life now. She took her wedding vows seriously and she has been a caregiver to me from the moment I sustained my brain injury. She has never treated me any differently and she always treats me with kindness and respect. Sure, there are days that she is pushed to her limit. Who wouldn't be? Being a caregiver is a full-time job. You don't get vacation days or holidays off. She wears the title of caregiver proudly and she takes her job seriously. Sheila is proactive in knowing things that I can handle and things she knows will throw me in a complete tailspin. If we are at a restaurant and I am having a really bad day, she knows it and will ask me if I would like for her to order for me. She has seen firsthand how bad it can get when I attempt to order and I can't get the words out. The harder I try, the worse it gets, and she eventually must step in and explain to our waiter or waitress why I am struggling. And, of course, we are always met with compassion and understanding.

I have seen firsthand just how much Sheila does. Things she shouldn't have to do, and I know it wears her out. She has had to take on some of the things I used to be able to do around the house. It must be a relief when I am having a good day, and I can take some of the burden off her shoulders. I have said it from the beginning, and I will continue to say that caregivers are unsung heroes. If you have never had to be a caregiver to someone, I promise you it's more work than you think it is. I am sure she worries more about me now when I leave the house without her. Trust me, I don't often do that, but I am sure she still worries about me.

We sat down with a digital recorder and just had a long conversation from her point of view. I knew there were things that I was leaving out, things that I had not written down or just don't have any memory of happening. Sheila has an amazing memory. I call it a blessing and a curse. She doesn't forget anything like birthdays, anniversaries, or people she hasn't seen in 30 years. She remembers events that happened and most likely the date and time they did happen. It's the most amazing thing I have ever witnessed. These are the things she had to say:

I'm not going to lie, the hardest thing for me to accept was you were no longer the person I married. I don't mean that in a bad way at all. You used to joke all the time and you were never serious. Now you are the exact opposite. You joke a little more now than you did early on, but you still are not the same person you were. It took a long time for me to accept that you had changed. I still loved you with all my heart, but I had to learn to love the new you.

The biggest struggles I've seen in you are your memory issues. The things you do remember you say happened yesterday. You might say we went somewhere yesterday, and we hadn't been there in months, but in your mind it happened yesterday. There are times that you will make breakfast on the weekend and a few hours later you will ask me what I want you to fix for breakfast. You have no memory at all of eating just a few hours earlier. I must remind you constantly of all the family members who have passed. Your Aunt Rena passed away a few months ago and not even a week went by before you were talking about her as if she were still alive. When I reminded you that she had passed away and we went to the funeral, you had no memories of it whatsoever. You also wished another aunt who passed away not even eight months prior a happy birthday on her Facebook page. This is a constant struggle that you deal with the fact that we can't seem to get to stick in your memory bank.

I've also had to take on more responsibilities in making doctor appointments or anything business related. You get confused and have trouble communicating your thoughts to the person on the other end of the phone. I always make sure I am nearby to step in if needed to help the person on the phone understand what you are trying to say.

When you get tired, I can always tell that your brain needs a break. Your words come out wrong or you stutter badly. Sometimes the words that are coming out of your mouth are not words at all. They are more like sounds or resemble words. When that happens, I have learned that you have totally exhausted your brain and it's time for you to go rest.

You always do your best when you are in a structured routine. During the week when you are working there is much less confusion going on. Once the weekend hits and that routine is no longer in place things get very interesting. Things get put in places they do not belong. I've found your cell phone and EpiPen in the refrigerator. Just last week I found a jar of peanut butter in the refrigerator as well. Things always run better when we have structure. It takes very little variation from that to throw you off your game.

And now you know why I love Sheila so much, she keeps me in check always. She does it in a loving manner. Sometimes I don't perceive it that way, but at the end of the day I know everything she does or says to me is because she loves me so much. She would move heaven and earth for me if she had the ability to do so. I can't think of anyone in the world I would rather have fighting on my team than Sheila. If I could turn the hands of time back and start my life over, knowing all the pain and heartaches, I would do it all over again, only if I had the promise that I would spend the rest of my days with Sheila by my side.

I wanted to share how Sheila and I met to show you a perspective of how our life has changed since my brain injury. Sheila took on the role of caregiver very early on in our marriage without knowing it, by helping me get through the baggage of my past. One thing you should know about me is I never dated. And mostly yes it was because of my childhood and not wanting to put myself into any sexual relationship whatsoever. For that reason, I never really sought out a girlfriend. I used to work as a ride operator at an amusement park that was inside a mall. I had made a lot of friends when I worked there and leaving them was the only thing I missed about my job. I had no social life outside of work, so once I got off work at my new job, I would stop by the mall to hang out and socialize with my former coworkers. One day a lady I was close to, she was like a mother to me, was training a new girl on how to operate the mini train. I approached her, said hi to her, and she replied, "Well hello Rob, let me introduce you to Traci. Rob, this is Traci. Traci, this is Rob. Do you know anyone who would like to go out with Rob?" I was horrified and embarrassed that she put me and someone I didn't even know on the spot like that. Traci answered her and said, "I do know someone I think would be a good fit."

People have been trying to fix me up with someone my entire adult life. I don't know what happened that day, maybe it was because I just got tired of people trying to find me someone, but I told Traci to bring me a picture of this girl, and if I think she is even half way good looking then maybe I will meet her. To be honest, I had no intention of meeting this person no matter what she looked like. I just had no interest in having a relationship at all.

A few weeks had passed, and I had forgotten all about being put on the spot like that. On my way home I stopped by the mall like I always do, and I saw the lady who put me on the spot at guest services and she was smiling ear to ear. I thought maybe she had gotten a promotion or something exciting had happened. As soon as I walked up to the counter, she said, "Boy do I have something to show you!" She laid a photograph face down on the counter. She told me this was the picture of the girl Traci was going to introduce me to. And then she said, "Now before you look at the photo, I want to remind you that looks are not everything." I was a bit relieved and thought, *Well, this won't be happening for sure.* I said, "Are you kidding me? You are trying to fix me up with a dog?" And then she turned the picture over and there she was. The most beautiful woman I had ever laid my eyes upon. I was in love with a picture, and we hadn't even met yet. I am not sure how long I stared at the photo before she said, "Um, well?" I said, "Sure, I'll meet her." I kept that picture and I still have it to this day. She was so excited and got on the phone and told Traci to make it happen. What Traci hadn't told us was she had not actually talked to this girl in years. If I had known that I never would have agreed to meet her. I am so thankful that information was withheld from me.

They arranged for us to meet at the carousel two weeks later. I ended up at the mall 30 minutes early. I have always been an early bird. If I am not at least 15 minutes early, I consider myself late. I decided to walk around a bit before we met. While walking around I ran into my old supervisor, so I walked up to say hello. "Hi Beverly," I said. "Would you like to see a picture of my future wife?" Beverly was all smiles and said, "Why yes, I sure would." She looked at the photo and said, "Oh my she is beautiful, where did you both meet?" I looked at my watch and replied, "At the carousel in about 30 minutes." She looked puzzled. She said, "You mean to tell me you haven't even met her yet?" I said, "No, this will be our first meeting." She handed the picture back to me and said, "Well she is beautiful, but you might not want to spring marriage on her during your first date."

After I was introduced to Sheila, we sat in the food court with Traci and chatted for a while. We exchanged phone numbers and we agreed to talk and see how it goes. We talked every night for the next three nights for at least two hours at a time. I really enjoyed talking with her, but I hadn't yet told her about my past. On the third night we talked a bit and Sheila spoke up and she asked if I was going to ask her out or what. I told her, "Yes, I would love to ask you out." We laugh about that now, but I am lucky she wanted to go out with me after that.

I wanted to take her somewhere nice on our first date. I had learned that she had never been to an Outback

Steakhouse. So it was my plan to take her there. She was excited to go there, I didn't tell her at the time, but I brought my entire paycheck with me, just in case she was a big eater. I mean, you never know. And this was my first date after all. The date went well, and we both had a good time. At first I didn't notice that our waiter only had one arm. How I didn't notice this is beyond me. Probably because I was so nervous being on my first date. How I came to know he had only one arm was when he brought the meals to the table, he seemed like he was struggling a bit to hand me my plate so I said, "Hey, let me give you a hand with that." Once I grabbed the plate and saw he was missing his arm I felt about five inches tall. I had put my foot in my mouth. Now he could tell by the look on my face that I was horrified by what I just said. That was so insensitive of me, and I would have never said that if I had known. He mouthed to me without Sheila seeing that it was fine. He knew I meant nothing by it, but I sure did feel bad. Years later when I tell that story, Sheila swears she never caught it. Our first date turned into several others. I finally got the courage to ask her to marry me and of course she said yes. I had no doubt in my mind that she would say yes. We'd already acted like a married couple almost from day one. The only thing she did not know was that I knew before we ever met that she was going to be my wife.

Shortly after we started dating, I would wake up in the middle of the night with the worst pain in my chest and my back. It would hurt so bad that I had to be taken to the ER and then sent to my primary care doctor for follow up. They told me I had acid reflux and to take medicine and I should be fine. But after a few weeks I would end up in the ER once again. The only way I could get any relief from this pain was to stand in the shower and get the water as hot as I could stand it, and just let it hit me on the chest. For a few moments I was relieved until I had to get out of the shower. This would continue to get worse as the weeks went on. The longer I dealt with the mystery issues the worse it got. I just knew at any point Sheila would give up and say she didn't want to see me any longer. Maybe she thought I was crazy. She never said that to me, but that was the narrative going on in my head. When things escalated and I ended up in the ER twice in one week she said enough is enough. Both Sheila and my mother cornered the doctor and advised him that something was missing. I was in too much pain, and this had gone on long enough. They refused to take me home until someone got to the bottom of it.

The ER doctor told them that they couldn't just keep me there all night, but if they brought me back in the morning, they would run more tests on me. The next morning Sheila took me back to the hospital and I had to do the test where they give you the thick liquid to drink.

The nurse told me to pretend it was a milkshake. It was the worst milkshake I ever had, and I nearly didn't keep it down. After suffering in pain for almost two years, we finally got answers. It was my gallbladder and it needed to come out as soon as we could get it scheduled.

As someone who was finally in a relationship, my surgery was scheduled for the worst day ever: February 14, 1997, or as you know it, Valentine's Day. I had other plans for that day, plans I made months before… it was the day that I was going to ask Sheila to be my wife. I didn't want to propose from a hospital bed, and I sure didn't want her to say yes out of pity. The big proposal had to be postponed until after I got the surgery behind me, and I was back to my old self again.

I had a very good surgeon who had the best bedside manners you could ask for. Sheila was there for me every step of the way. Thank God she was, because after we went through registration and had to wait to be called back, she asked me if she could read the papers I was given. After reading for only a few seconds she jumped up and said come with me, we are going back to registration. They have made a big mistake, and sure enough they did. They had me down for brain surgery. I was already a ball of nerves, and this did not help. I was so glad Sheila was there to catch that mistake!

Sheila made sure I was very well taken care of. She came by every day after she got off work to check on me. She brought me meals and kept me company until my parents got home from work. If there was anything I wanted, she would have gotten it for me. She has always been by my side and has been my biggest cheerleader and protector. There is never a day that I don't thank God that he put her in my life. I often feel I don't deserve to be loved as much as she loves me. Many people have questioned me before as to why I make that statement. That is a hard question for me to answer. I have thought about it at length before and questioned myself why do I feel so unworthy of love? I honestly believe that it's a combination of the mental abuse that I received from my mother when I was growing up compounded with the sexual abuse as well.

Those two circumstances are how my life began and set the stage for me to feel unworthy. Those points in my life are what instilled in me that I am more of a burden than I am a blessing. So now that I am nearing my 50th year here on earth, I can say with confidence that 90% of the time I finally feel worthy of love. I am human and I definitely have my bad days. I am just so thankful that I have a wife who can love me for who I am and not who I could be.

After I proposed to Sheila, and she said yes, we decided that we needed to start saving for a house and for a wedding. Sheila was always better at saving than I was.

I wanted nothing but the best for her, so I would always spend my money on her. She broke me of that early on or we would probably not be where we are today. One thing we both agreed on was that we would not live together until we were married. Sheila told me she wanted me to live by myself in the house we bought a year before our wedding. She knew I needed to be out of the situation I was in living with my mom. Even as an adult making my own money and paying my own bills my mom was still trying to control me. She would tell me that I couldn't buy things she didn't approve of. She would tell me what time I needed to go to bed and when I needed to get up in the mornings. I agreed with Sheila and told her I thought it was a great idea to move into our house as well.

One morning about a week before we were to close on our house I was in my bedroom watching TV. I couldn't have even been up an hour yet. The door burst open, and my mother poked her head in the room and she stated, "I just wanted to let you know that I never wanted you. You were a mistake. I was on birth control when I got pregnant with you. I never wanted you." She slammed the door behind her as she left. I laid in bed wondering what in the world I just witnessed. I hadn't even talked to my mother that morning. I was in pure shock that she felt the need to let me know how much I wasn't wanted. The closing date could not get here soon enough.

The beautiful fall morning finally came when we owned our house. We couldn't wait to rush to our first home together. As soon as they handed us those keys, off we went to our empty home. *Our* empty home. We began making calls to get everything turned on. I was working a late shift, so it was no problem for me to be home during the day as people came to install services. Sheila worked not even a half mile down the road, and she came home for lunch every single day.

The day the gas company came to turn our gas on is a day that I will never forget and I still thank God to this day that I am here to tell the story. The man was on time and got the gas turned on. He asked me if I ever used a gas stove, and I told him I hadn't. He gave me a quick five-second tutorial of how to operate it and then he was on his way. I went to the living room and started watching TV for a while before I had to get ready to go to work. Not long before it was time for me to leave I began feeling nauseous. I started to call Sheila at work to tell her I wasn't feeling well. I picked the phone up and I couldn't remember her phone number. I was getting really confused out of nowhere. The only thing I could think of doing was to call my supervisor. I told her how I was just fine a few moments earlier and now I feel so sick to my stomach. When I told her I tried to call what's her name and she said do you mean Sheila? I said, "Yes, that's her name." She became worried about me. Things were just not right she would tell me later. Somehow, she managed to call Sheila at work and tell her she needed to get home, something was wrong with me. Sheila let no grass grow under her feet, she was there in record time. As soon as she opened the door, she said, "OH NO, Rob you need to get out of this house right now." The smell of gas just about knocked her down at the door. I had not noticed it because I had been exposed to it all day long. I had no idea how lucky I was until she came to my rescue. That was a close call that could have had a very different ending. I am so thankful everything worked out.

That was a real teachable moment! It's important to never take for granted warning signs. Looking back all of the red flags were there. I made the assumption that the professional who turned on my gas would have known that there was a leak somewhere. Being a new homeowner I would have never known to check anything out after the fact. Whether it be a gas leak or anything else in your life, remember that life is precious, and we only get one chance to live it. So never take one day for granted. I tell everyone that a life lived in fear is a life not lived. And I do strive to practice what I preach. I don't always hit the mark, but I have a much better track record nowadays. It is great to go with the flow and live in the moment. Just make sure whatever you do, you use wisdom and ask someone who knows more than you do. This will take you far in life.

I promised myself from the day we met that I would do everything in my power to make Sheila happy. Trust me when I tell you I am not perfect, and I fail miserably daily. But the effort is there, and she does know that. I tell her all the time that I would crawl through glass for her. And I do mean that, she is my everything. She has been by my side through my best days and through my worst days. I could not ask for a better partner to spend my life with. I have always talked highly of her to anyone I have conversations with. I call her my bride even to this day. There is nothing that she wouldn't do for me, and there is nothing that I wouldn't do for her. We are a team, and we stand strong through all the storms of life.

I hope everyone finds their Sheila. It brings me so much joy when I hear stories of how couples take their vows seriously. Realistically, not every day is a bed of roses. But if you find the person who has your back no matter what, those bad days don't seem so bad. When you find the person who God intended for you to be with, the small stuff doesn't seem worth arguing over. Life feels so complete when you have someone who really will love you through sickness and health. If I never found my person, I would have never done the hard work of getting help when I needed it. My life would have looked much different than it does now. I am able to be a better version of myself because of who she is. Marriage is hard work, but worth the effort. It makes you so thankful to be alive when you have the right person standing by your side. Things you never dreamed you could do suddenly become possible. Experiences that you may have never had are a reality. I would live my life over a hundred times again, as long as I was able to spend my life with my wife, my best friend. I shared events that happened to me during the early part of my marriage to help you see how unexpected life is. Just because you get married, that doesn't mean you will never have your ups and downs. Not every day is a honeymoon for sure. Learning to get through the bumps in the road will make you appreciate the good times even better. Appreciation in my opinion is a gift. Appreciation means that you see the full value of something's worth. It makes us more humble and helps us to enjoy the human experience with full intention.

BEHIND CLOSED DOORS

It is important to give some background on my mother, even if it is a bit selective, before I dive headfirst into my earliest memory of trauma. I know my mother loved me, but she had a hard way of showing it. In many ways I feel that she was carrying so much baggage from her own childhood that she wanted to make sure the world knew who was in charge, and it was her. She ruled with an iron fist, and you had better do as you were told, or it would not go well for you. She was also OCD to the point you had to clean up your toys the very second you were done playing with them, or when she felt you were done. On one occasion, I must have been in kindergarten, I was playing with my toys in the middle of the living room floor and I left to go to the bathroom. When I got back a few moments later all my toys had been bagged up and taken out for the trash, just because I hadn't cleaned up before I went to the bathroom first. That is just a very small glimpse into the tin soldier life I lived growing up.

My mother was very controlling, it was her way or the highway. People walked on eggshells around her up until the day she died. I know my mother loved me and I believe that how she treated me while I was growing up was a direct result of the way she was raised. I heard my mother say she wanted better for her kids than she had. And she was generous to a fault. But you did not want to be on her bad side. The best thing you could do is agree with her – because at least then it was much more peaceful. My mother was very controlling and would fly off the handle at the snap of a finger, which made me guarded with anything I would share with her. I remember when I was in my third grade Christmas play. I feel like we were rehearsing for the musical *Cats* as much as we had to practice. At the end of one of our rehearsals we were going back to the classroom, the teacher stopped in front of the bathrooms and instructed us to go to the bathroom if needed, and if we were thirsty to form a line single file to get a drink out of the water fountain. I was a shy kid and was never first to do anything, so I waited for the other kids to get in line before I did. I ended up at the very end of the line. When it was my turn, I walked up to the water fountain and bent over to get a drink. I pressed the handle and it was at that moment the teacher grabbed me by the arm and jerked me away from the fountain. She took her hand and smacked my rear end hard. It stung for what seemed to be hours, even though it was probably only three or four minutes. The teacher said, "That was for showing off." I have never talked back to a teacher in my life, but I looked at her and asked her, "What did I do? I was only getting a drink of water." She told me I knew what I had done, and I needed to get my act together. To this day I honestly don't know what on earth I did to warrant that discipline.

I had made up my mind that I was not going to tell my mother what had transpired at school that day. I knew if I did, she would yell at me and then probably yell at the teacher. This ate at me all day and into the night. At bedtime I went into my mother's room, and I told her that I wasn't going to be able to go to school the next day. She asked me why I couldn't go, and I said because tomorrow I am going to be sick. The real reason was I was ashamed of what I might have done to get into trouble with my teacher. In my mind I had really done something wrong, I just didn't know what I had done. My excuse for being sick in advance didn't land well with my mother. She knew something was wrong because I loved going to school. I had never faked being sick. The questions started flying: Why don't you want to go to school? What did you do wrong? It was a nonstop interrogation until I finally cracked and told her what happened. She asked me if I was showing off and I told her I had not been. I did exactly as I had been instructed by the teacher. My mother knew I wasn't lying. I was the kid who threw himself under the bus and would rat *myself* out from guilt if I didn't tell the truth to begin with. Of course, this was the fear of God she had instilled in me practically from birth.

The next morning, she woke me up earlier than normal and told me to get ready because we were heading to school. It would be at least another hour before school started. I had a gut feeling that things were about to go from bad to worse for me, and I was right. By the time we got to school it might have been 30 minutes before class started. My mother was practically dragging me down the hall by the hand. She was on a mission; I just didn't know what that mission was. We got to my classroom and my teacher had her back to us and she was writing the day's lesson plan on the chalkboard. Without any hesitation from my mother, she blurted out, "Who in the hell do you think you are to lay a hand on my son, you mother #$@** Bi**H." The teacher's hand flew across that chalkboard and the chalk went sailing across the room. I was totally horrified at what just happened. My mother chewed her up and spit her out. All the while getting closer and closer to the teacher. I really thought I was going to start seeing my mother drug away in handcuffs at any moment. But somehow, she didn't lay a hand on her.

After my mother finished with the teacher, she grabbed me by the hand and went down the hall to the principal's office. She announced that she was there to see the principal and the lady behind the counter told her that he wasn't in yet. My mom walked behind the counter and said, "Which one is his office? I'll wait." The principal, having heard the commotion, stuck his head out of his office and said, "Hello can I help you?" My mother said, "You sure can." And proceeded to tell him what happened the day before. She left out the part where she almost beat my teacher up. She told him she wanted me out of her classroom today. The principal told her he would be glad to switch classrooms, but we are about to go on Christmas break, and he thought it would be best if we did the change after I return from break. My mother told him she thought it would be best if she just went down the hall and knocked the teacher's teeth out. More words were exchanged between the principal and my mom. At some point the principal figured out that he was fighting a battle that he wasn't going to win. He told my mother to take me home for the day and to come back 10-15 minutes before school started the next morning and he would have everything worked out and me in a new classroom. My mom was happy with this resolution and that is what happened. She was happy and that's all that was important to me. When my mother wasn't happy, there was no chance of me, you, or anyone being happy, period.

The next summer we moved, and I was more than happy to leave my old school and friends after the show my mother had put on. But more importantly I was beyond excited to move because that meant I would no longer have to cross paths with the person who hurt me the most in my life, my abuser. This was a new start and the only potential obstacle in my path would be my mother. She took me to school on my first day. It was raining cats and dogs that day. She made me wear a bright yellow raincoat. I would fit in, I was told. All the kids are wearing them. I may have spotted one other kid dressed as if they were heading out to sea. Other than the fact I was dressed like Gorton's Fisherman, the day went very well. The school was totally different from what I was used to.

Everyone met in the center of the room, and we sat cross legged, and then broke off into units each morning. We had four teachers in each grade, and we would rotate to learn a new subject. The teachers were wonderful and I only had my guard up with one teacher. She appeared to be a teacher who was always looking for someone to make a mistake so she could pounce on them. I made sure that when I was in her class I was on my extra best behavior. I was able to stay well off her radar almost the entire school year. The last week of school we were in the lunchroom. I can't recall the main course in the hot lunch line, but I know we had baked apples and peanut butter balls. The reason I remember this so well is I had just sat down with my plate, and I picked up the plastic fork and placed it in the baked apples. They looked so good, and I was ready to tear it up. As soon as I poked my fork into one of the apples, the prong of the fork broke and went flying across the table. I looked at the person next to me to see if by some chance they happened to pick up an extra fork, and they had not. I thought I would just go back up to the line and get another fork. Before I could even stand up, the teacher I had avoided all school year came up to the table and slammed both hands down in front of my tray. She leaned in and said, "Young man, pick up your tray and follow me." *Here we go*, I thought, *she finally found something to make my life miserable*. She walked me to the trash can and said, "Throw the plate away." I looked up at her and said, "But I haven't been able to eat any of my lunch yet." She pointed to the peanut butter ball on the plate, and she told me to pop that in my mouth and dump the tray. She then made me stand in the corner for the entire lunchroom to watch me the whole lunch hour. I nearly choked on the peanut butter ball, but I dared not say a word for fear she would just make my life even more miserable. The desperation I had for even just a drink of water to get that dry cotton mouth feeling to go away. At the time it felt like torture, nothing to eat but a peanut butter ball and no water to wash it down. It was going to be a long day.

We lived two blocks from the school, and I ran home as fast as I could that day. I was starving and couldn't wait to find something to eat. As soon as I walked in the door I went to the kitchen and my mother was stirring whatever it was she was cooking. I told her I was hungry and how much longer till supper. She laid the spoon down on the stove top and asked me why I was hungry. I never come home from school hungry, so something was up. I assured her nothing was up, and I was just hungry. My mother wasn't buying it. The interrogations had begun, and I knew I was fighting a battle I wasn't going to win. I told her what had happened at school. She reached over and turned the stove off, grabbed me by the hand and said, "Come on, we are going to talk to the teacher." She was walking what seemed to be 60 miles per hour down two blocks to the school. I had taken my shoes off and was barefoot and I can still feel the heat of the pavement on my bare feet. We arrived at the school and the doors had already been locked. I thought: *crisis avoided.* But my mother was not going to let a locked door stand in her way. She began to pound on the doors repeatedly to the point I thought the glass would surely break. She kept this up until eventually a janitor happened to be walking down the hall to take out the trash and he came to the door and let us in.

She began walking down the hallway and at some point realized she had no clue where she was going so she asked me where in the bleep was my classroom. I pointed down the hall and off we went again. When we got to the classroom there were still three teachers standing there talking. To protect her identity, I will refer to her as Mrs. Smith. My mother walked up to the first lady and said, "Are you Mrs. Smith?" It was like a scene out of a movie because that teacher, who happened to not be her, and the other teacher both pointed to Mrs. Smith. My mother got in her face and laid into her. She kept leaning in closer and closer and Mrs. Smith kept leaning back further and further. How she didn't fall to the ground is beyond me. It was funny. The other teachers were doing their best to not laugh their tails off. My mother told Mrs. Smith she wanted my lunch money back for the day since her son didn't get to eat any of his food because of her. Mrs. Smith advised my mother that she would need to go speak to the principal. They don't give refunds on lunch money. My mother then advised Mrs. Smith that she had better dig deep in her pocketbook and fast, or she would reach in through her rear end and pull a dollar and change out herself. With that she took option A and grabbed her purse and pulled out two dollars. I think Mrs. Smith was expecting change, my mother grabbed the money, said thanks, and then grabbed me and said now let's go talk to the principal. Luckily the principal was still in his office so we were able to resolve the issue immediately. If she had to hold that anger in overnight, it would have ended in an even bigger blow up. My mom laid into him next. She told him the whole story and advised him that she was taking me out of school for the remainder of the school year. I think we had two or three days left to go anyway. He agreed it would be best as well, given how upset she was, and he didn't want there to be any fear of retaliation towards me for my last few days. I was so thankful that I didn't have to show my face back there again. I would have the summer to recover, and hopefully everyone would forget and move on.

Earlier in my life an incident happened that gives you another insight into my mom. I was five years old and I shared a bedroom with my older brother. We were lying in bed one night at bedtime and we were giggling and telling each other funny things, as brothers do. My mother sent in my dad the first time to tell us to be quiet and go to sleep. We were quiet for maybe two minutes and then the giggling and laughing began again. This time my mother showed up at the door. My side of the bed was closest to the door, so I was the first to be snatched out of the bed. My brother was told to come with her as well. He got to walk; I was drug down the hall to their bedroom. My mother then proceeded to grab a roll of duct tape from her top dresser drawer and rolled it around my wrists and my ankles and sat me on the floor. She did the same to my brother. She turned the light off and lay on the end of her bed and shined the light on us and dared us to even make a whimper or she would give us something to cry about. I knew this was not something a mother should do to their kids. I would spend the rest of my life asking myself why she would treat us this way. Why did she have kids if all she can do is treat us this way? I loved her because she was my mother, and she gave me life. But I held such a grudge towards her my entire life for the way she treated me and my brother. She was always much harder on me for some reason. And there were times in my life that out of nowhere she would just tell me that she never wanted me, and I was a mistake. That word mistake has always haunted me. All my life I have felt that I am not worthy of love, not worthy of life, and I bought into the lie that I was a mistake. I have worked through that lie, but it took nearly 40 years to get to the point that I have accepted that I am not a mistake. Yes, maybe it wasn't planned, but I am not a mistake.

There were happy memories and I know that she did the best that she could to show me that she loved me. It seems strange, but her yelling at my teachers was her way of showing love. I tried hard to give her the benefit of the doubt. Even though I am not a parent, I do see the struggles other people have trying to raise children. One thing that never set well with me growing up is that she held me and my brother to the same standards despite our age difference. My brother is seven years older than I am and we fought all the time. With that big of an age difference, we really didn't share a lot of common interests. When we would get into an argument we would both be punished severely. I don't think we shouldn't have gotten off scot-free, however someone that much older than you should know better and the punishment shouldn't be nearly as severe for someone who doesn't know any better.

Looking back, there were so many teachable moments that my mother would have benefited from. I think more people would have attempted to offer friendly advice to my mom, but chose to keep their mouth shut to avoid the wrath that would follow. I recall many times my brother would get a mere smack on the wrist so to speak and I would be grounded for a month. The punishments in our home never seemed to fit the crime. It would leave me so confused growing up as to why she was so severe with me and soft on him I can only speculate that he did get his fair share before I was ever around. Unlike me, he was never afraid of my mother. He would stand up to her in a heartbeat. I can recall many times the argument got so heated that I thought someone would call the police. In all the years growing up and talking back to her, he always got away with it. He didn't seem to cave to her threats of being grounded or whatever the punishment may be. I can only remember one time in my life that my dad ever stepped in and became vocal. My brother was so angry at my mom that he reared his fist back as if he were going to hit her. Out of nowhere my dad lunged across the room and pinned him against the wall. I can't tell you verbatim what was said, but he drove the point home that you will never in his presence lift a hand towards his wife. He must have really made his point clear, because I never witnessed my brother come close to raising a hand toward her after that day. Once he was old enough to drive, he came and went as he pleased and he would not give you the luxury of knowing where he would be and when he would be home. That was not the same outcome I had when I began to drive. I had to give details of where I was going and when I would be home. This was just the way things operated in our home. There was never any rhyme or reason as to what rules applied and when. When I moved out of the house to live on my own, she started acting like a mom for the first time in my life. I will admit that for the longest time I would be very cold towards her. I carried so much resentment for the way she treated me growing up. It was a constant struggle with my emotions. I loved her because she was my mother, but I resented her so much. How could she not see that what she did to me hurt me to my core? I had to remind myself often that I no longer had to live in a state of constant pain. I didn't have to walk on eggshells around my mother any more. Once I fully accepted that I was free from the pain that my mom would put me through, I was finally able to breathe a sigh of relief and really begin to live my life.

I believe with all my heart that she sensed the tension between us in my adult years. She tried to buy my love with gifts. I could never say I liked something, or she would buy it on the spot, even though I told her not to. I would fight her tooth and nail until I gave in and let her buy it, or she would go behind my back and surprise me with it later. Eventually I would stop commenting on things I liked so she didn't do that for me. I didn't want her to buy my love. It was never for sale, and it still isn't. I just wanted what everyone wants and that is to be treated with kindness and love. I missed out on so many years of my life without receiving that, I fear that I am guilty of not giving that out as freely as I would have liked to. This has resulted in my making every effort I can to ensure people feel loved and accepted. I strive to hit the mark 100% of the time, but I am human and I am sure I may fail every once in a while. I only hope that people don't think I do that on purpose.

Getting to the point of acceptance wasn't something that happened overnight. It was when I began doing the work of healing from my childhood sexual abuse that I was able to find my own self worth. Once I was able to finally let go of the emotional baggage I discovered that my life did have meaning. There are people in my life who truly care that I live and breathe. People accepted me for who I am and not what they felt I should be. I finally forgave myself for allowing me to be stuck in a tiny box that had no room for anyone else in there with me. After I made that breakthrough with the help of my counselor, I finally decided it was time to forgive my mother for the pain that she had caused me all my life. I had to teach myself that forgiveness doesn't mean that you are letting someone get away with their bad behavior. It means so much more to me now, it means that I acknowledge that you may have caused me pain, but I am allowing myself to not be affected by your words or actions. It means that I no longer give someone else the power over my life to control my happiness. Let me tell you, it is so freeing to say I forgive you. Saying those two simple words – I forgive – releases the chains of the heavy burdens that you are carrying. It frees your heart and soul to have more room for love and happiness. I know it sounds too simple to be true. Holding a grudge only hurts the person looking in the mirror. When you hold a grudge, it is something that is eating at your mental well being constantly. It does more harm to your health and wellness than it will ever do to the person who you harbor resentment towards. I have had to remind myself several times since I made that realization, that forgiving doesn't mean I am giving someone a free pass to harm me. It gives me the ability to heal from my wounds and the power to keep pressing on.

I don't want you to get the impression that every day of my life was filled with heartache and sorrow. I do still have very happy memories that pop into my head even to this day. When we moved from the home where the sexual abuse happened, I met our new neighbor and he would be my best friend for years to come. His mother would take me on every family vacation they went on. She treated me like her own son and I am forever grateful for those relationships I built back then. It really kept me grounded and helped me to have the childhood fun that I was robbed of. From fifth grade until he moved away during our high school years we were inseparable. We both became almost like brothers, but ones who liked each other.

OVERCOMING INTIMIDATION

I imagine at some point in your life you have come across a bully. Whether on the playground in school or someone in your professional career that pressures you to do things that may blur the line of ethics. According to a recent study it is estimated that 1 in 5 students ages 12-18 are bullied. The percentage of cyberbullying has more than doubled from 2007 to 2019. There has been a decrease in the number of reported cases and has continued to decrease each year. I believe the only way we can make progress to keep that going down is continued education. Our schools are doing a much better job than ever before. Even though we are doing better as a whole, there are so many new ways to bully now than there were 20-30 years ago. The internet has exposed us to cyberbullying, mainly because people are able to hide behind a screen name. Somehow it gives them the fuel they need to say whatever thoughts come into their head. What I have learned in my adult life that I wish I had known as a teenager is if someone is attacking you, take a stand and let a teacher know what is going on. If a teacher will not listen to you, take it to the school principal. There is no shame in reaching out to ask for help. Many believe that will only cause the attacks to continue or increase. I have found that once you call someone out for who they are, they become exposed and have to come face-to-face with the fact that their actions are not acceptable. Most will be embarrassed that they let what they conceived to be all fun and games cause harm to someone else. Others may try to seek revenge and make your life miserable. But the good news is, once you have brought attention to a teacher or principal, they will be able to have your back in case a retaliation should be attempted. Bullies are only as strong as we allow them to be. Once you strip away the ammunition they use to attack you with, they are powerless. I do hope that you consider these words of encouragement as you read further of my experience and how I wish I had this insight when I was younger.

In work situations it would be wise to address the person bullying you in face-to-face conversation in private. By doing so, this will take away any type of embarrassment to that person or give them a reason to put on a show for the crowds. I have found that many people are more reasonable when they are being talked to in a calm fashion. It could be that the person doing the bullying has no idea that is what they are doing. So that would prevent a scene, and the issue was handled in a calm manner. Should you be met with confrontation. I would quickly end the conversation and at that point you should talk to your immediate supervisor or manager. Most workplaces nowadays take bullying very seriously and will shut it down fast. As long as you go through the proper chain of command the issue will be addressed and eliminated.

When I was in the sixth grade, I had a bully. I had never drawn attention to myself and I had a very small group of friends. Had it not been for them I am not sure if I would have had the will to go on. They were my rocks. I have since lost touch with them, but I often wondered how they are doing now. Where did life take them? First semester went off with no hiccups at all. Once I got into the second semester is when a bully entered my life.

I never once said or did anything to this person to make him retaliate against me. But I don't think bullies wait around for someone to ruffle their feathers. I guess I was just an easy target and probably someone he knew he could get away with picking on. It didn't start off big at first. He would walk by me and "accidentally" knock my books or papers onto the floor. He would announce that I had dropped something and laugh. This was the first time I had a bully in my life. I didn't want any part of it, but we don't get a say in that when someone sets out to make your life hell. He sat in the seat right behind me in math class and every chance he had to throw something at me, smack me in the back of my head, or tie my shoelaces to the feet of my desk when the teacher wasn't looking, he took it.

He would get to class seconds after I did, maybe he did this on purpose or perhaps it was just something that just happened. Either way, he would immediately come up to me and begin picking on me. This happened the entire nine weeks I shared a classroom with him. I recall one day he came in and got in my face and started calling me fat boy; I never said a word. Then he began saying things to me like, "I know you are a fag. Is that who you are, are you a faggot?" It made him mad when I would not respond to his insults. Then he'd start pushing me on my shoulder. I think his intention was to knock me out of my chair, but he was not successful. He continued making derogatory statements to me and despite my best attempts not to, I began to cry. This is clearly something you don't want your bully to see, but it happened. It was at that moment that the teacher walked into the room. I was so glad she did! She noticed that I was crying and asked me if I was ok. I made up some excuse and she told the bully to please take his seat. To this day I really feel that she knew exactly what was going on. I am glad she didn't draw more attention to it, I think that would have just made the situation worse. However, I am also mad that, as an adult, she would turn a blind eye to someone in need. As an adult, you would think the right thing to do would be to address the situation. But turning a blind eye is never the answer.

The bully would continue to take shots at me for the remainder of the semester and I took it like a wimp. Some would probably argue that I empowered him by not saying anything. Maybe I should have gone to an adult and let them know what was going on. Things were a lot different back then than they are today. It seems that the worse you were back then, people just allowed that kind of behavior to continue to avoid confrontation. At least that is the way it was at my school.

I got lucky in my next two years in middle school and never shared a class with him again. It was either by chance or maybe the teacher who never spoke up to the bully had gone on my behalf to the counselors and made sure that I never shared a class with him again. Either way the situation eventually worked itself out. It didn't make the pain I'd gone through any better, but at least I never had to deal with the situation again.

During Christmas break of my freshman year of high school my cousin asked me if I had heard that my bully had been in a car accident and died. I hadn't heard the news. Human behavior nags at you that you should feel horrible that he passed away. How can you not feel grief from the passing of another human life right? Especially a young one. My emotions were in a total war. Should I cry? Should I rejoice that the man who tortured me daily in school could never again be a threat to me or anyone else? The only thing my mind would allow me grasp was all the hard times he caused me in middle school. I could feel no sorrow for him at all. I wanted to so badly, but I felt sorrow for his parents. I knew they loved him and most likely they never had a clue he was the class bully. I have to give them the benefit of the doubt that their son wasn't a total monster when he was at home. It stands to reason that when you are around friends you act totally differently than you would act in front of your parents. Although I never knew his parents, it is very possible that his home life wasn't a bed of roses either. Maybe I was an easy target for him to get his frustrations out on. For days after I found out he had passed I wondered if he had changed his ways. Did he grow out of that phase of his life? I wrote a backstory in my head that he never bullied anyone ever again. He was going places and had a bright future awaiting him after graduation. Maybe he would be a counselor to help people who are facing bullies themselves. I put myself through this for weeks. I think deep down I was trying to put my bully on a pedestal that he didn't belong on. No story I created in my head was going to change what he had done to me. Once I finally accepted the fact that I couldn't make him something he wasn't I began to feel relief. I never reached a point where I felt sorry that he had passed away. I hope I do someday, and perhaps the more I work on my healing, the more I will allow myself to feel sorrow for him. I do feel bad that he is gone, I don't want anyone to die like that. I do hope he changed though. I hope he made his parents proud and his absence from this world is one that cannot be filled. I recently had a discussion with my counselor to try to come to terms with why I could never feel sorrow for his loss. She made a really good point that made so much sense. We live in a society where we speak bad things about people, but once they die we build them up to be something they were not. If someone is a horrible person and they die, their status doesn't change. Death doesn't come with a magic wand that undoes all the hurt and wrong that someone has done all their life. While it is very sad when someone passes away, how we view that person should not change. We feel we paint a picture that doesn't exist for our own benefit. That really helped me get past that feeling of feeling guilty for not being sad. Sometimes it's ok to just be ok. And there is no "should" in how you process *anyone's* death, especially a past bully.

Somehow, I managed to avoid any additional major traumas until I was in the ninth grade. I can remember approximately when this happened because it was the week of the derby. There were many celebrations locally that lead up to the Kentucky Derby each year. It was a busy week. I took the bus to school when I got to the ninth grade. It was too far for me to walk. When I got off the bus that afternoon to go home like I did every day I noticed that there was a car that had started following slowly behind me. I felt my heart beating faster but I did not want to draw attention to the fact that I was aware I was being followed. I'd seen too many TV shows where people get kidnapped. At one point I thought maybe I was just overreacting. Who would want to kidnap a teenager? I have never made any enemies so surely there was no one trying to retaliate against me. But still I had a sickening feeling in my stomach that something bad was about to happen to me. I started to walk just a little faster but not so fast that It made it appear that I was on to whoever was following me. I had just two more houses to go to until I got home.

As I reached my house I began walking through the yard towards the front door and the car came to a stop and a man jumped out and began walking towards me. He stated his name, which I do believe was a made-up name and flashed a badge really fast and put it back in his pocket. At this point I reached the front door, and I had a death grip on the door handle. The "cop" said he had reports of someone going door to door selling things in the neighborhood and asked what I had in my bag. I told him I had just gotten off the bus from school and I had my school books in the bag. At this point my heart felt like it was going to jump out of my chest. I kept hoping someone in the house would see me and think, why was he talking to a stranger and come inquire. But then it dawned on me, it was supper time. We always ate as soon as I walked in the door. I could have been standing there with my hair on fire and no one would have noticed. With my death grip on the doorknob, everything about this situation did not feel right. I didn't believe this man was a police officer for one second. As the man was talking, he was moving closer to me and my fight or flight was kicking in big time, so I opened the door and I yelled "DAD, come here for a second, this cop wants to talk to you." I could see the expression on the man's face change drastically. My dad came to the door and the man began to tell him that he had received numerous complaints about people going door to door selling books in this area and that I had fit the description. Obviously it wasn't me as I'd just gotten off the school bus. He told my dad if he saw anything suspicious to just notify the police. Then he said to have a nice day and got in his car, and he left in a hurry. I told my dad how he started following me the moment I got off the bus, and how he had approached me and everything about the situation felt wrong. He agreed that something didn't seem right about the whole ordeal, so he called the police department and let them know what had just happened.

He described the man and the car he was driving and told them the whole story. The police officer told my dad that it was not illegal to sell door to door, so the whole story didn't add up. He told him that there were no plain clothes detectives driving that make and model of car and he advised us to come file a police report. The office told my dad to have me pay close attention to my surroundings in the days ahead. They felt that I may have been followed for a while and to just keep my guard up. I felt so violated. The emotions flooded back into my mind and soul, the feelings that I had felt when I was sexually abused as a child just washed over me like a tidal wave. Suddenly I saw the face of my abuser, I could smell the cheap aftershave lotion. I felt like a deer in the headlights. I felt short of breath and I could feel my heart pumping faster. What were this man's intentions? All the emotions from my childhood abuse came rolling back into me like the flood gates had just blown open. I couldn't sleep at all that night. Every time I heard a car drive by the house, I was convinced it was him coming to get me. Any time I heard a noise big or small I quickly jumped out of bed and peaked out the window. I had become a prisoner in my own room. I was constantly looking over my shoulder. The next day I told a good friend of mine what had happened. I was terrified to walk to the bus stop by myself anymore. He told me not to worry, starting tomorrow he was going to come to my house every morning and walk with me to the bus stop. Safety in numbers, he said. He lived four houses down from me, so it wasn't that out of his way to come to my house every morning and walk with me to the bus stop. He had the biggest heart of anyone I had ever known. He is the guy who would literally give you the shirt off his back. He probably will never know how much that gesture meant to me. His kindness has never been forgotten. We have lost touch over the years, but every time I run into him, that is the first thing that pops into my head. Everyone needs a friend like him in their life.

I was always the first one on the bus after the bell rang in the afternoon and I had become pretty good friends with the bus driver. His name was Bob, and everyone loved Bob. He was a soft-spoken man and you could talk to him about anything, and he would listen to you like you were the most important conversation he was going to have all day. The next day I talked to Bob and told him what had happened. I told him how scared I was to walk home from the bus stop by myself in the afternoon. I didn't even have to ask Bob, he told me that starting today he would be dropping me off at my front door going forward. I wish everyone had a bus driver like Bob. He was a people person but more importantly he had compassion for people. I thanked Bob every day for weeks for going the extra mile, he didn't have to do that. One day he laughed, and he said,

"I am responsible for making sure you get to school safe and back home safe." Basically, he was telling me, look, I am just doing my job. I wasn't used to people being nice to me on purpose. I am so thankful to have had someone in my life who did their job and kept me safe.

For several weeks there was a car that would drive by our house slowly at night. Sometimes he would keep going, sometimes he would park a few doors down and sit in his car for several minutes before driving away. After a few months had passed by, the car stopped coming. Life started looking normal once again, but it would be several months before I finally got over that trauma. Nothing bad happened to me, but it felt personal, I felt violated, I felt taunted and harassed. Whatever the guy was looking for he didn't get. But he left me emotionally vulnerable for a very long time.

I didn't have another run-in with what I perceived to be a would-be stalker until much later in life. I had just started a new job in a call center to answer calls about dental procedures. People would call in to get an estimate on how much a root canal or an emergency extraction would cost them. They may be out of town and having a dental emergency and they would call in to have us locate a dentist that would be close in proximity to where they were located. The training for this position was a six-week course and the binders we trained out of weighed about 10 pounds, they were so thick. I felt like I was going to be a dentist by the time I finished training. It was stressful to me when I was offered the position that under no circumstances was I allowed to miss even one day of training, should that be the case don't bother coming back. They put the fear of God in you to be on time and you had to pass the course to keep employment.

I can't recall how far into training I got before the following incident happened to me. I do remember that we were going to be reviewing the past week's information to study for a big test. It was a sunny day as I drove to work that morning. It was a peaceful drive because for the longest time I was the only person on the highway. I had the radio playing my favorite songs and I sang right along with it. I had at least 10 minutes left in my drive before I would arrive early so I could sit in the break room and enjoy peace and quiet before I had to start learning some more information that I probably would never have to use.

As I was passing an exit, I noticed a white van getting onto the highway behind me. It's important to note that I am never one to speed. If the posted mileage said 65 you can bet I was probably doing 64. I had passed the exit without the need to accelerate to allow room for the white van to safely merge into traffic. I did move over to the fast lane as a precaution, my thinking is typical drivers always go much faster than they need to, and he would surely pass me moments after getting on the highway. I noticed there was a ladder on top of the van, so my first thought was it was a business van, maybe heating and air, or a roofer. Sure enough, as I suspected he sped up to pass me. At least that's what I thought he was going to do. As soon as he met up with me, he stayed right next to me going the same speed I was going. It is important to note that I am a person who tends to be paranoid. Given my past history of abuse it stands to reason that I have real trust issues and immediately go to the worst case scenario. And so me being immediately suspicious of the intentions of the driver in the white van makes sense. I slowed down just enough for the van to get ahead of me. My plan was to then get behind him to avoid that awkward feeling. But as I slowed down, he did the same. I glanced over and I noticed there were two people in the van. Since it was becoming obvious that he wasn't going to speed up, I decided to speed up to get in front of him. Either he would stay behind me, or he would get frustrated and end up passing me. As I sped up, he did the same. Eventually he slowed down and got behind me. I felt relief until I looked in the rear-view mirror and noticed he was on my bumper. I sped up and so did he. I switched lanes and he followed pursuit. Forcing me to go faster and faster. He ended up in the fast lane and that's when the passenger rolled his window down and I could see he was yelling but I didn't know what he was yelling at me. He began to throw empty coke bottles and trash out the window hitting my car. At this point I was in fear of my life, they clearly had some kind of a motive and I didn't see this ending in a positive way. Against my better judgment I did what I felt was the only way to get out of the situation. I began accelerating to speeds I had never driven before. The last time I looked at the odometer it was kissing 90. I had to get away from the people harassing me. My thoughts were if I end up dead it's not going to be because two people with nothing better to do decided that today was the day to pick a random driver to torture.

I managed to get off the exit where my training class was, and I was still driving very fast at this point. Just as I was making my turn in the parking lot I gave my rear-view mirror one last glance. I didn't see the van, but I wasn't taking any chances either. I quickly found a spot where a lot of other cars were parked, and I sat there watching my rear-view mirror for any signs of the white van. I sat there not even 10 seconds before I saw the van coming down the road slowly. It was obvious they were trying to find me. As they went past and out of view, I jumped out of my car and ran for the building. I walked into the lobby and took a seat at the break tables and just sat there quiet as a mouse. I had to walk past the security guard, and he must have figured something was up. I tried every morning as I entered to tell him good morning. Sometimes we would chat for a second or two, but then I would take a seat until training. I walked past him that morning and said nothing at all.

One of my coworkers showed up a few minutes after I sat down. She started talking and I didn't hear a word she said. I knew she was talking, but it was no more than the Charlie Brown teacher to me at that point. I have no idea how long she talked before she finally said, "Rob, Rob, ROBBBB, are you ok?" And that is when the waterworks began. I broke down and it was hard. My body was shaking so hard I was in near convulsions. My coworker jumped out of her chair and ran over to me to console me. I was hyperventilating and it just wasn't getting any better. Someone ran to a Coke machine and purchased a soft drink to try to calm me down. The trainer was the next person to walk in the door and she saw the commotion and quickly came over to find out what was happening. She was able to calm me down, she had such a still, calming voice. She sat down next to me and told me to take my time. She asked the rest of the crowd who had gathered to go ahead to the training room, and she would talk with me.

Once my audience was just down to the trainer I began to calm down. She told me to take my time and explain to her what the problem was. I walked her through the whole story of events of what had transpired with the white van as it had unfolded. As I began to give her more details of what I had just been through, she put her hand on my hand and nodded at the appropriate times, giving me the look of approval that I needed, just knowing that my feelings were justified was starting to make me feel better and safe. She asked me if I would like to go home for the day, she didn't think that I would be able to learn anything anyway. I told her I needed my job so I would stay. She assured me that I would not lose my job. She told me things come up that are beyond our control, and no one would be in trouble. She strongly advised me to make a police report. I told her yes, I want to do that. She went to the security guard and asked if he wouldn't mind calling the police for me and letting her know when they arrived so she could come back to be with me.

The police showed up 10 -15 minutes after the call was made. I ran through the whole story once again with the police officer. I gave him the best description that I could. It is hard to get a good look at someone when you are driving as fast as I was. I asked the police officer if I would be in trouble for driving over the speed limit and he chuckled and he told me if he was in my shoes, he would have probably gone even faster than that. He assured me I was fine, and they would be on the lookout for the van. He told me for the next few weeks he would patrol that part of the highway at that time of the day. After the police report was made, he asked me if I would like to have someone come to get me. I told him I would rather just drive home.

I didn't want to be here any longer. He said that was fine with him, but he insisted that he follow behind me for a few miles, just to be safe. I agreed to those terms, and we were on our way. It made me feel so much better knowing that he would be keeping a look out for me. Sure enough, the next day when I went back to work, I saw him sitting on the side of the highway. He had kept his word.

I came to the conclusion that there are people in this world you can depend on. We may feel that no one cares and just when we feel like we are down for the count. Someone shows up for you. There is so much to be said for that officer who probably could have been doing something more important than sitting on the side of the road waiting for me to arrive at my training without being afraid of what is around the corner. But he did exactly as he said he would. He was a man of his word. I wish now that I would have gotten his name and thanked him for making me feel safe in a world that I felt was against me. I am sure his response would be, "I was just doing my job." But little did he know that by doing his job and taking his oath to protect and serve seriously, would have a lasting impact on me all these years later. My advice to you the reader would be to never miss a chance to thank someone in the now. Never leave an opportunity on the table to let someone know the impact they made on your life. You may feel that it is small, but you will never know how a kind word can potentially go a long way with a stranger. I suggest that you never know when you may make a friendship that will last a lifetime over a simple moment of gratitude.

Also, remember to be good to other people any chance you can get. Hold the door open for a stranger, tell people to have a great day, smile more, and tell people they matter. Sometimes all another person needs is just to know someone cares. In my case just knowing someone cared enough to lend a listening ear and show compassion made a world of difference to me. It reminds me of a sign that I am sure many of you have seen before "Be kind, everyone you meet is fighting a battle you know nothing about."

LETTiNG GO

In 2015 my mother had to undergo her second heart valve replacement surgery. She somehow got an infection that the doctors had no idea how she got it. It was explained to us that when you have a foreign object in your body, like a heart valve, when you get an infection in your body, it will attack any foreign objects first. The infection had pretty much destroyed that valve requiring her to have the second surgery. This infection was nothing to play with. It required her to have six weeks of antibiotics through an IV. My wife and sister-in-law took turns taking care of her, administering the shots she had to take. We feel strongly that this would have been caught sooner, but she was working a job for a doctor who should have retired years ago. He is the kind of doctor who has patients jam packed in the waiting room willing to wait to see him because they knew he would prescribe whatever it is they needed. He did not take care of my mother and her condition worsened. She was admitted to what I will refer to as a mini hospital. It was a facility that was started by a few doctors. The quack doctor admitted her there because there was no other hospital in the area that would now longer allow him to see patients at their facility. To spare you a long story, we had fought to get my mother to a well-known hospital that could treat her condition better. He fought us for four days before I got involved and had to move mountains to get him to release her. Once he agreed to release her he told the nurse to give her antibiotics before calling an ambulance to transport her. I found out later that he knew the infection had returned four days earlier and he chose to do nothing about it until we got him to agree to move her. After she went to the next hospital, she was seen by the best doctors. They did everything they could for her. They did a great job keeping us updated. The original plan was to get her heart better and if that couldn't be achieved they would discuss putting her on a transplant list. With each passing day her condition declined. The day finally came that the doctors had to tell us there was nothing more they could do. I remember it like it was yesterday. My brother and my dad were not at the hospital. My Uncle and his wife were there with me visiting my mother. The heart doctor walked into the room and asked if he could speak to me outside in the hall. When the words came out of his mouth, I knew this was it. This is when they tell me it's over. We got into the hall, and we found a small quiet hallway where he could tell me what the next steps would be. They had found that she had a brain aneurysm and that was the least of their concerns. When a doctor tells you that a brain aneurysm is low priority, you know they have done all they can do. They had tested her heart that morning and it was past the point of no return. He told me he would be calling hospice to speak with us that afternoon. He put his hand on my shoulder and told me how sorry he was that he didn't have better news to share with me and he went on his way. As soon as he turned to leave my eyes filled with tears and I could still feel the warm tears running down my face. I was trying to hold it back as best as I could, but there was no fighting it. My aunt had stepped out into the hallway and listened in to what I was being told. She could see how emotional I was getting so she went back into the room and got my Uncle Tim to come be with me. I didn't have to say a word. The look on my face told him all he had to know. I suspect that he already knew when the doctor pulled me into the hall. My Uncle Tim helped me get my composure and I had to make the phone call to my dad and to my brother to tell them what I had just found out. I was running on autopilot at that point so I could not tell you what I said to them, nor what their reactions were to the news.

We met with the hospice nurse, and she filled us in on what the next days, weeks, or longer would entail. The only thing we knew for certain was we could not take her home to die. The condition she was in required three nurses to even help her out of bed. We didn't have the manpower nor the money to pay for around the clock care. None of us had the luxury to take weeks or months from our job. And my dad wouldn't have let us do so if we wanted to.

We had to break the news to my mother and that was probably one of the worst days of my life. The hospice nurse gave us pointers on what to say and what not to say. We wrestled with who should speak first and who should be in the room with her when we told her what we had found out. We felt it would be best if she didn't have an audience surrounding her as we told her there was nothing else that could be done. My dad and I discussed the fact that her sister who was really fighting us to send her home should at least be included. She had been at the hospital every day since Mom was admitted and we didn't want her to feel excluded. Somehow the decision was made that I would start the conversation off. I wasn't fond of that idea being the youngest but I agreed. Once we cleared the room, we all sat there for what felt like an eternity. I think we were all hoping someone else would say something, anything. The longer we sat there the more paralyzed I felt. I knew what needed to be said, but I could not bring myself to let the words leave my lips. Finally my brother spoke up and said, "Mom, so we have some news to tell you and I don't know how to say it." That was all she had to hear, she looked at my Dad and said, "I'm going to die aren't I?" Dad didn't say a word, but tears began to fill his eyes. She then looked at me and asked, "How long do I have?" And with that the water works began. She began wailing and sobbing so loud that it sent chills up my spine that felt like a million knives. She kept saying she wasn't ready to die yet, there was so much living she wanted to do. She kept saying this isn't fair, this isn't fair. And I must agree, it wasn't fair. Here was a woman who growing up made my life a living hell. The same woman who took great joy in embarrassing me any chance she would get. But the last few years she tried her best to be mother of the year. She made sure to call often or invite us over for supper. At times she was a little over the top with the way she would tell everyone she came into contact with that I was something special. Something she never did when I was a child. It seemed that she was trying to make up for so many of her mistakes in raising me. I know she had a good heart. Who knows why she treated me the way she did. But she was still my mother, and I wasn't ready to see her go either. Facing reality and in such a short period of time wasn't the news I wanted to hear nor was I emotionally ready to feel those emotions. I had to come to terms with the fact that someone who I loved, yet who drove me crazy would soon be gone. My mind became so clouded with fear, and not even things that I would consider normal. My first fear was I would forget her voice or her laugh. I made sure I got videos of her so I could still remember those sounds. Even though I have recordings of her voice, there wasn't anything to laugh about at this point. I never did get to record the distinctive laugh that she had. Oh how she would crack herself up at her own corny jokes. I always told her that she was her best audience. We would spend the next month or so in the hospital. Visiting her every day and spending as much time with her as we could until it was time to say goodbye.

One night before we went to the hospital, Sheila asked me if I had planned to sing at the funeral. I told her there was no way I could do that. I have sung at many weddings and funerals in my life, but there was just no way I could find the strength to sing at my own mother's funeral. Once we got to the hospital that day, Mom was having a decent day. There were some days that you would think she was about to jump out of bed, put on her clothes, and say let's go. I learned from the hospice nurse that when someone is near the end of life, they will get surges of energy and then go right back into a point that they could go at any moment.

When we got to my mother's room, I sat down in the chair next to her. She began questioning me about how my day had gone. Did I have anything good to eat? Then she grabbed my hand and out of nowhere she said, I want you to sing at my funeral. I looked at Sheila and her eyes got big. I looked at her because I thought maybe she had said something to my mother and I could tell by the look on my wife's face, that wasn't the case. I looked at my mother, lying in her bed not knowing if we had a day left with her, a week, or a month. All I knew was there was no way I could turn down my own mother on her deathbed. If she wanted me to sing the star-spangled banner, I would have. I told her I would be honored to sing per her request.

The time was drawing near, the last few days she lay still in her bed non-responsive to us. She was just there. We knew it was down to hours or days until we would lose her. I was really praying hard that she didn't pass on my wife's birthday. I didn't want to ruin her day, but it was looking more and more possible each day. The day before her birthday my mother was in a coma, and it seemed clear it would only be a few more hours to maybe a day or two. I decided to stay the night with her. My wife and brother said they would be up in a few hours, and they would stay the night with me as well. When I got to her hospital room, she was the only one there. It was getting late, but I decided I wanted to sing her one more song before she left this world. She loved to hear me sing so that was the least I could do for her. I shut the door to her room to try to keep the noise down. I pulled the chair up close to her bed and I told her I know you can hear me, so I wanted to tell you one last time that I love you. I am going to sing you a song now, I know it won't even compare to the wonderful sights and sounds you will behold soon. But for some reason you love my horrible voice, so I get to torture you with it one last time. I chose an old song titled *Search Me Oh God*. I think I chose that because it was always so beautiful and moving to me. I know that had to make my mother so happy.

My brother showed up and shortly after my wife. The nurse brought us a cot to sleep on in the room. But we never slept. We talked all night and into the morning. Talking about all the memories we had growing up and later in years. Occasionally one of us would doze off for a few minutes. But we quickly regained where we left off. 4:00AM came around and I just wanted to get away for a few minutes to go home and take a shower. I wasn't gone very long and on my way back to the hospital I stopped to get some donuts for us to snack on. We didn't have anything to eat, and I knew they would appreciate the jester. I got back to the hospital around 5:30AM and Mom was still holding on. The mood had changed in the room. Most likely because we were so tired. It got really close to 6:00AM and my wife decided to step out into the hall to make a phone call. I was seated to the right of my mom and my brother to her left. We both just sat there in silence for the next few minutes. For whatever reason, we both turned and looked at my mother at the exact same time. I saw her take her final breath and be birthed into her new home. I whispered to my brother "that's it." He asked me if I thought she had passed and I said yes, that was it. I walked to the nurse's station, and I said my mother just died. They went into her room, checked on her and confirmed that she had passed away. It was expected, yes, but it still hit me hard. Reality had just smacked me in the face, and I didn't like it. I did have comfort to know that my mother was a Christian and I knew where she was at now.

We talked to the nurse and told them we would like to go home to get my dad. We did not want to break the news to him over the phone. He had stayed home and was in the process of getting ready so he could come to the hospital to be with his wife. The nurse told us to take our time and to go get my dad so he could come say goodbye before they took her body. I was in no shape to drive, and neither was my brother. Sheila was always so good in a crisis. She told us that she would drive us to go get my dad. We stopped along the way and picked up my brother's wife so she could be with us as well. I went into the house first and dad was walking down the hallway putting his shirt on. He told me he was just about ready to go. I told dad I had something to tell him, and I didn't know how to say it. He looked at me and I could already see a tear forming in his eyes. I said, "Dad, mom passed away this morning." I had never seen my dad cry, I think back to all the funerals over the years we had attended, his mother, his dad. Nothing ever seemed to move this man to tears. But that day I saw my dad cry for the first time. I told him the nurse said it would be ok for us to bring him back to the hospital to say goodbye. Other than having to tell my mother she was going to die, this was the second worst day of my life. I can't imagine how it feels to lose a spouse. I pray that I never have to know that feeling. But we all know that life is short and one day rather we like it or not, we all will face that day.

I'd like to interject briefly here about my dad in order to give you a small insight into what influence he has had in my life. Growing up I was much closer to my dad than my mom. Dad was a man of few words. I alluded to that in the eulogy I gave at my mom's funeral... Dad spoke when he had something to say, and mom spoke until she had something to say. Dad has always been soft spoken, which is probably where I got that trait. His passion in life was bowling, and he would probably bowl seven days a week If he could. My mom always said if she went before he did, he would probably miss the funeral if it were on a bowling night. To this day I think she got the last laugh because the day of her funeral happened to fall on one of his bowling days.

Since mom passed away, he has really changed. The man that used to be of few words, has no issue coming up with things to talk about now. I can't help but think that he never really had a chance to get a word in while mom was alive. But I do find it humorous but also nice to see that he does have something to say. Dad just turned 80 this year and he is still working part time, bowling as much as he can, and living his best life.

Grieving the loss of a parent, especially when that person was mentally abusive, is undoubtedly a complex and challenging experience. It's normal to find yourself in a space where you're mourning their absence while also dealing with the weight of the harm they caused you. It's crucial to acknowledge that their abusive actions don't diminish the sadness you feel or invalidate the complexity of your emotions. It's okay to feel a mixture of sadness and relief simultaneously. It's completely normal if you're not okay with everything right now. Remember that healing doesn't happen in the snap of a finger, and it looks different for everyone. For many people you may feel guilty, I know I sure did. When you notice a sense of guilt, remember that this does not mean there's anything wrong with you, or that you are remembering things wrong. Guilt is a natural reaction for survivors, and many times simply acknowledging and validating its existence can be freeing. Guilt does not invalidate your experience. It is okay to feel a range of different emotions during this time. There is no right or wrong way to experience grief, especially the death of someone who was harmful towards you.

When grieving an abusive relationship, you may unexpectedly discover some positive aspects. Dealing with grief can lead to profound realizations about your own strength and resilience. It can become an opportunity to reclaim your narrative and focus on your healing rather than dwelling on the hurt. This process opens doors for personal growth and allows you to form healthier bonds moving forward. You may uncover hidden aspects of yourself that were buried under the pain, enabling you to set boundaries and practice self-love. Now I don't get the chance with my mom to resolve it.

Remember that there's no rush in this process. It's okay to take your time and navigate through your emotions at your own pace. Surround yourself with people who support you and understand the complexities of your journey. You deserve to experience and process all the emotions that come your way. There's no right or wrong way to grieve. Take care of yourself, prioritize self-care, and be gentle with yourself throughout this healing process.

The healing process comes back full circle to forgiveness. Forgiveness serves as a powerful catalyst for healing and closure, allowing individuals to release the burdens of resentment and anger. By choosing to forgive, one can foster emotional well-being and restore inner peace, ultimately leading to a sense of liberation from past grievances. This process not only mends relationships but also promotes personal growth, enabling individuals to move forward with renewed strength and clarity. Embracing forgiveness can transform pain into understanding, paving the way for a healthier, more fulfilling life.

DEEP WOUNDS

Abrain injury may have been what started me on the path of personal healing, but what I realized is that the array of traumas I experienced over many years of my life is what really needed healing. I've been carrying baggage for as long as I can remember. Many things I didn't even realize. I became an expert on putting situations away on a shelf to try to hide the trauma from my brain. But, as you might be aware, whether you deal with your issues or not, they are always manifesting in various ways. One coping mechanism I leaned on heavily was food. Food was the one constant that never failed to comfort me. Which is why I was always the chubby kid. Food was the constant in my life that I would turn to in order to deal with my emotions, both good and bad. A result of me being an overweight kid, was the increased friction between me and my mother. She was constantly shaming me for being overweight. She would force me to be on diets and take diet pills. That only caused me to retaliate by eating even more. I would sneak food after my parents went to bed. I would take every chance I had to shove food in my mouth. That wasn't a wise strategy, but that's what I did and there is no way to change that now. My mother said she was concerned about me being overweight for health reasons, but I believe the main reason is that it embarrassed her. My mother was a person who loved to fat shame. She would go out of her way to say how fat someone was. Her "go to" insult for anyone always began with "you fat..." followed by even more derogatory statements.

When I was around seven years old, she was obsessed with making me lose weight to the point that she ordered diet pills out of a catalog. She referred to them as my fat pills. I hated the word fat with everything in my soul. I wasn't on those "fat pills" very long before my grandmother learned that my mother was forcing me to take them. I had very rarely heard my grandmother raise her voice, but this was one time she did. She really laid into my mother until I thought Mom was going to cry. She was the one and only person I know who was able to stand up to my mother and get away with it. My grandmother was the nearest and dearest person I could count on. Don't get me wrong, I have lots of relatives who I know would give me the clothing off their back if needed, but my grandmother gave me a special kind of love I've not felt from anyone else.

The earliest childhood trauma is one that is the elephant in the room. According to the U.S. Department of Health and Human Services, Children's Bureau: 1 in 5 girls and 1 in 20 boys will be a victim of sexual child abuse before they turn 18 years old. During a one-year period in the U.S. 16% of youth ages 14-17 had been sexually victimized. Children are most vulnerable to child sexual abuse between the ages of 7 and 13. My assault happened when I was six years old. I spent almost an entire lifetime living a life filled with guilt. I had reasoned myself into believing that had I just stayed home that day, none of this would have happened. Sure, it may be true that if I'd stayed home that day it would not have happened. However, this young man was nice and never made me feel uncomfortable when I was around him. He was a trusted friend of the family, a next-door neighbor, who I visited often. So had it not happened that day, it was surely bound to happen another day.

I remember going to his house that day, just as I had done many times before. I walked on in because that's just what we did back then. He greeted me with a smile and suggested that we go to his bedroom to play. I didn't think anything of it, as his mother was in the living room . I figured he didn't want to bother her while she watched TV.

He was a high school student, so I have questioned most of my life why his mother didn't have a problem with him playing with young kids when there were much older boys to hang out with in our neighborhood.

When we got to his room, he shut his door and locked it. I honestly didn't think that was strange. He had never done that before, that I can recall. I had no reason to think anything bad was going to happen just because he did that. He asked me what game I would like to play. I thought about it for a few seconds, and I spotted Twister on his game shelf. I hadn't played that game before, and it looked like it might be fun. He told me that he had just got it and it was really complicated and it required several players. I don't know if that is true or not, because I have not played Twister to this day. So, I told him he should pick a game. He went to his dresser drawer and pulled out these plastic rope-like things. I really don't know what they were or what they were called. The closest I could come to describing it would be if you had zip ties that were about an inch wide.

He showed me the plastic ties and asked me if I liked playing cops and robbers. What six-year-old boy doesn't like to play that game? I told him I sure did. He suggested that I had just robbed a bank and he was going to catch me and handcuff me. He opened his closet door and said, "Now you hide in there and when you come out, I will catch you and put you in jail." Into the closet I went and waited for my command to bust out of the closet, which in my pretend world was the bank I was robbing.

"Come out with your hands up," he yelled. That was my cue to exit the 'bank.' I did as I was instructed and came out proudly holding my hands up. He grabbed me by one of my arms and threw me on his bed. He told me this was my jail cell, and I would have to stay there until I learned my lesson. He paced back and forth in front of the bunkbeds for a minute or two, and I started getting bored being in jail. I told him this isn't fun anymore, let's play something else. He sat down on the bed next to me and he said, "Well, I have an educational game we can play." He looked at me and asked me if I thought I wanted to be a dad someday. I told him I guess so, but I would have to get a wife first. He asked me if I knew how babies were made. I told him the stork brought them, that's what I had learned from the cartoons. He laughed and he said, "That's all fake. I can show you if you want to know." I told him that sounded ok to me. He told me I had to lie down on his bed, and he would show me. I did just that, I had no idea what was about to happen to me. As I laid there, he took his pretend handcuffs and tied one arm to the bedpost and then the other. At this point I was thinking this doesn't seem right. The mood felt different. I started to feel scared, and I didn't understand why I was feeling that way. Then he unbuttoned my jeans and pulled them off me and it was at that point he did the unthinkable to me.

Once he completed the act, he gave me a very stern talk. He asked me if I understood what had just happened and I told him I did. But I really didn't understand. All I knew was I did not like what he had just done to me. He said, "What you just did is illegal and if you tell anyone you will go to jail." He continued, "Do you realize if your parents find out what you just did, they will never love you again?" Everything he told me was what I had done. I believed with all my heart what he told me was true. He had totally convinced me that everything that had just gone down was my fault. I had asked for this, he made sure to remind me that this was all my idea. I wanted to know how babies were made. He totally brainwashed me and I felt immediate shame. I told him I needed to go home; I was sure supper was probably ready. He reminded me once again that if I told anyone, I would be locked up for the rest of my life.

I walked home slower than I normally would have. I didn't want to go home, but I knew I didn't want to stay at his house either. I can remember stopping at the end of the driveway and thinking, how could I let this happen? And how do I hide this from my parents? I knew my mother would totally kill me if she knew what I had just let happen to me. I also knew my mother had a short temper. She would have gone next door and killed him for sure, then *she* would be in jail, and I would never see her again. There was no way to win. I was so ashamed of my actions, and I planned to keep this a secret I would take to my grave. To this day I have never told my parents or anyone in my family what happened that day. Mostly because of the embarrassment of saying what happened to me. No one ever knew until I was put in a situation when I was 19 years old. I was working at an amusement park in a local mall called River Fair Family Fun Park. I started as just a ride operator, but I did other jobs as well. The best part of my job was being a mascot. The River Fair mascot was two dogs called Hooper and Hannabelle. I was Hooper. When I first signed up to be the mascot, I wasn't 100 percent sure that I would be able to do it. I had a hang up with hugging people. I would let my grandmother hug me all day long, but I would avoid other people like the plague. It seemed like such a fun job that I wanted to at least try it. It turned out to be so rewarding. Yes, the kids all ran up to me and wanted to give me a hug, but somehow when I had that costume on, that was like a mask to the outside world. It was like my security blanket. It would be such a wonderful experience that I would gladly do again if given the chance. I went to baseball games, the dream factory, and I did commercials for the fair. It was my cup of tea.

One Friday I was contacted by my supervisor, and she asked me if I could work on Saturday. I normally didn't work on Saturdays, but we were short staffed, and as those who know me know that the word no is not in my vocabulary. Naturally I agreed but asked if I could do something that wasn't so stressful. I would later regret asking for such a favor. Soon my entire safe world would come crashing down.

I was put on the golf course; it was a simple job so that was fine by me. Everything was going smoothly, and I made it through half of my shift before I saw him – my childhood abuser who I had not seen since I moved away was standing 20 feet away from me. I totally panicked and I grabbed the telephone next to the cash register and lay on the floor of the golf house. I didn't know if he saw me, but I did not want any dealings with him whatsoever. I called my supervisor and used a tone with her that she had never heard before. I will refer to her as Tina to respect her privacy. I said, "TINA GET HERE NOW!!!" She asked if something was wrong, and she could tell by the tone in my voice there was. I did not have time to explain what was going on. I felt like my heart was going to jump out of my chest. I repeated once again, I need you here and I mean now. She got there in probably less than a minute, but it felt like an hour. She showed up with another supervisor and when she saw me on the floor, she thought maybe I had passed out or something was medically wrong. She rushed in and asked me what was wrong. I said I need to get out of here right now, this is not a joke. She helped me off the floor and the other supervisor took over my place as Tina escorted me to the break room.

We sat down at the table and another employee was finishing up their break. Tina could see the fear on my face, and she asked if I wanted to talk about it. I told her not really, but I am sure you are wondering why I just freaked out in front of God and everybody. She then patted my hand and said, "it's ok, take your time." I whispered to her that I would talk once the other employee finished their break. We sat in silence for the next 10 minutes. As I sat there, the memory of my childhood raced through my brain repeatedly. Reliving all that pain once again was too much to bear. A secret that I had kept to myself for the past 13 years was about to be let out of the bag. I began to ask myself if I could trust Tina with my secret. I felt strongly that I could, but what if she told one person, and then that person told someone. It would not be long before the whole world knew.

After the employee went back to their station Tina asked me if I was ready to talk, she asked me if a customer had done something to me, or was I being bullied by another employee? I told Tina that what I was going to tell her I did not want to go any further than from myself to her. She told me that I could trust her. I must have asked her a dozen times to please keep what I was about to tell her between the two of us. She swore that whatever I told her would never leave her lips. We sat quietly for a few more minutes while I got up the nerve to tell her what had happened to me. Then I relived, for the second time, all that trauma from my childhood. I gave her probably more details than she bargained for, but she let me speak without interruption. The shock on her face while I was speaking had me questioning myself. Was I doing the right thing? Did she really need to hear all these details? But I couldn't stop talking. The flood gates had opened up and I had to get it all off my chest. She was in tears by the time I finished telling her. She promised that she would never tell anyone what I had told her. She thanked me for calling her to help me get out of that stressful situation. She asked me why I never told my parents. She had twin boys, and she would want them to come to her if something like that ever happened to them. I told her how controlling my mother was and how she would have taken what happened to me and not only would she have probably killed the guy, she would have blamed me for putting myself in that situation to begin with. It was a no-win situation for me no matter what. She understood. I asked her what she would have done if something like that happened to one of her kids, and, without hesitation, she said, "I would have killed him." I was touched and also so surprised by the look in her eyes and how upset she was for me, someone she wasn't even related to. I actually believe she could have killed someone if they had done that to one of her boys.

Tina sat with me for the longest time and wanted to make sure I was going to be ok before she left me alone. She told me she wanted me to just stay in the breakroom for the remainder of my shift so I could get my composure. I did not argue with her at all because the last thing I needed was to go back to the floor and potentially come face to face with my abuser again. For the rest of my shift, I sat quietly in that uncomfortable plastic break room chair. I let my mind just go blank so I could shut the entire world out. The only thing I could hear was the faint hum of a fluorescent light bulb in the maintenance shop behind me. Other than that, you could hear a pin drop. I really enjoyed sitting there, having no one around me. I felt safe and I was ok with that.

I am not sure when I finally decided to be open with my best friend Jeff, but the day did come when I eventually found the courage to confide in him. We had been friends since high school. Jeff knew everything there was to know about electricity and woodworking. He was just a genius at anything he wanted to do. It wouldn't be long before we became best friends. We spent so much time hanging out together. He had always been there for me, and I was always there for him, so I felt like I needed to be open with him. I was so afraid that Jeff would think differently of me once I told him. He sat quietly in a chair after I let him know what happened. He began to shake his knees back and forth. He always did that when he was bored or when he had something on his mind. After a few moments he just stared into the distance and he said, "Rob, I am so sorry that happened to you. Thank you for trusting me and letting me know." He totally understood why I had never told my parents. He had witnessed the way my mother was, I didn't even have to explain to him my reasoning for not telling her. I am glad that I took the risk in trusting Jeff with my secret. It is so hard to be vulnerable, I feared that he would distance me and go his separate way after a while, but we are still best friends to this day. That was such a weight off my shoulders.

When I started dating my now wife, I told her as well. I felt that I could trust her, and I wanted to be up front and let her know what she was getting into. She couldn't have been more caring and understanding. Yet another reason I love her so much. I call her my angel; she is the best thing that ever happened to me. I came clean with her very early on when we were dating. She kept my secret from others as I had asked her to do. After we were married, she saw the nightmares I was having. That was something I could not hide from her. She encouraged me to get counseling to help me sort things out. And it was the best thing I ever did. I honestly think had I not, I would not be here today. My mind was really messed up from carrying that weight all my life, along with all the other traumas I had experienced in my childhood. Having gone through counseling and getting myself in a much better place has caused me to always encourage others to seek help. It never hurts to talk your problems out. The worst that can happen is you get better. And isn't that the point after all?

I won't lie to you, counseling is not something that you can do one time and poof you are cured. I like to compare it to an automobile. You must keep it in running order or it will break down on you. You must keep the oil changed and the tires rotated to keep it in shape. So yes, along the way, I have had to have a few pit stops to talk about the problems again. Triggers can come from anywhere and throw you back into a tailspin. It can be something as simple as a smell, the way someone might smile at you, and it can be a song that throws you right back into that moment. It is essential to recognize the strength within you as you navigate the journey of healing from childhood trauma. Embrace the progress you have made, no matter how small, and understand that each step forward is a testament to your resilience. Remember, it is never too late to seek support and to prioritize your well-being. You possess the power to redefine your narrative and create a future filled with hope and possibility.

CRIPPLING EFFECTS OF ANXIETY AND PTSD

One of the unfortunate symptoms that comes along with a brain injury is anxiety and PTSD. Some people think both are one in the same, but they are not. The primary difference between an anxiety disorder and PTSD is how the condition arises. Those suffering from anxiety can develop the condition due to stress or environmental factors, genes or biological, or sometimes unknown reasons.

People with PTSD, however, often experience intense anxiety and related symptoms in response to exposure to a specific traumatic event. PTSD symptoms can be triggered by virtually any situation in the lives of those suffering from it, but the situations are primarily restricted to those similar to the original traumatic event.

I feel it is important to address both of these situations because they have been a part of me from the moment I got my brain injury. To give you an example of how the PTSD has affected my daily life, I have noticed that any time I reach to open a door now, without even thinking about it, I push whatever arm is free in front of me as if to protect my head from further injury. For several months after my injury I had a lot of nightmares, each one reliving that moment of impact over and over again. It has made me even more scared of bees than I was before. Talking with a psychiatrist really helped me a lot. She was able to get me to a better place and got me the medication that was right for me. I haven't had nightmares for two years, but I do still keep my guard up whenever I open a door.

Therapy is something that many people are afraid of. They feel it makes you weak or that others will judge you for having to get help. I am a strong advocate for people to seek help. There is no shame in wanting to improve your life and get better. The only advice I would give people who need therapy is to do your homework. I would advise against just calling the first person you come across. Not every counselor is the right fit for every patient. If the person you are seeing isn't a good fit for you, you will not get the best care for your situation. As funny as it may sound, I had to shop around for a counselor when I was first married. Sheila is the one who pushed me to get help.

The first person I saw was probably 10 years past her expiration date. Her office felt like I was visiting my grandmother's house. I felt so uncomfortable talking to her about what happened to me when I was six years old. It was like cracking a walnut. I was so guarded. But the thing that threw me off the most with her was this tiny string of spit that hung from her lip as she talked. I could not tell you one thing that she said to me that day. As she was talking, I watched the string go from the bottom lip to her top lip, from her top lip to her bottom lip. Eventually I started counting how many seconds it would hang on the top lip versus the bottom lip. I kept watching the clock and wanted so badly to just ask her if we could be done with the session. Then my ADHD would kick in and I was back to counting seconds on the spit once again. Once my hour was finally up I was mentally exhausted yet I got nothing from the session. The counselor grabbed her book to make my next appointment. I told her I really had a lot going on the following week and I would have to check with my wife to see what days work best for her. I assured her I would call her back later to schedule my next visit. I have a feeling she wasn't holding her breath that she would hear from me again. As we walked to the elevator I told Sheila there is no way I can see this woman ever again. I told her what had happened, and the way I told her in very descriptive details had her in stitches. After she got her composure she agreed that If I wasn't going to get anything out of it, that it would be best if we keep looking.

My choices were pretty limited in our area. There were more men counselors than there were women. I have nothing personal against men, but with what I had gone through in the past I was adamant that I had to have a woman counselor to speak to. After a few more searches we finally found someone who was the perfect fit for me. This is why I tell anyone who is going to see a therapist to make sure they are right for you. Had I stuck it out with the first person I saw, maybe she would have helped me eventually. Perhaps I would have just gone through the motions and never gotten a thing out of it. Either way, I made a lot more progress by making sure that I found the person who was right for me.

As for the anxiety that I deal with, that is still a work in progress to this day. Medication has helped me tremendously, but there will probably always be a part of me that still will face that demon when it rears its ugly head. For the most part we have a plan in place and Sheila is great at seeing the warning signs beforehand. There are times that she will tell me something wouldn't be good for me because there will be too many people there. She has become a pro at reading situations and being a buffer so I can avoid the added stress and anxiety. The more anxiety and depending on the situation will lead to a full panic attack.

The problem, though, is that sometimes we can't predict what potentially might cause added stress and anxiety. A really good example is I had to have a tooth pulled last year. I have been to the dentist many times before, and I have had to have a tooth pulled before in my life. I knew the specialist who was going to do the procedure and it was not something out of the ordinary. Normally Sheila would join me on any appointments I may have in case she needs to speak for me or help me fill out paperwork. This particular day she was unable to go with me because of work .She made an arrangement with her Mom to take me and drop me off. Sheila would come pick me up after she got off work. We did everything we knew to do. She wrote out things that I would need to put down on the forms so I wouldn't panic. We had all of the bases covered. I didn't get lost going to my appointment and I even arrived early. I had no issues filling out the paperwork, because of the good notes that my lovely wife provided me with. Everything was going perfectly until they called my name and took me to the room. Once I sat in the chair I could feel my knees shaking. Then I started to feel my heart racing, I looked at the door and thought maybe I should make a run for it. That's when the dentist walked in the room and started telling me everything about the procedure and it was like listening to the Charlie Brown teacher. At that point I was just shaking and almost in tears. He tried his best to calm me down, but there was no calming me down. He handed me the form that I needed to put my signature on and my hand was shaking so bad I couldn't even write my name. He finally told me to just put an x down and that would be sufficient. Somehow he was able to give me the shots to get me numb. I was hoping that would calm me down, but no such luck. The entire time he was pulling my tooth, his nurse held my hand and kept telling me I was a champ and everything was going perfect. I thought if I am being a champ I would hate to see how your cry baby patients act. Once everything was over he read me a list of things that I knew I would never remember. I was able to make it to the reception area to pay and they asked me to sit in a chair behind their desk. They must have seen this in patients before because they told me I was about to pass out. I remember handing the lady my wallet and saying take what you need. I still think that's funny to this day. How she knew what card to charge is beyond me, but everything worked out fine. Someone called Sheila to have her come pick me up and she told them she was actually on her way and not far from the building. One of the employees knew there was no way I could safely walk to the car on my own, so they grabbed a wheelchair and proceeded to take me downstairs. I kept apologizing to the lady the entire elevator ride down and I explained to her that I have a brain injury and it causes me high anxiety. She was so kind and told me I had nothing to apologize for. She explained to me that she knew what I was going through because someone in their family had a brain injury. As bad as I had felt for causing a scene, it really wasn't something that any of them had never been witness to before. And it's very likely I wasn't the worst patient they had ever dealt with either. It's funny how when we are in the moment and panic is in full force things are never nearly as bad as what we think they are. After the dust had settled and we had time to think about what had happened, Sheila came up with a plan for the next time, if there ever is a next time. She said if we ever have to go through this again, we will pay to have you put under anesthesia to avoid that again. That plan was something that really calmed me down and makes me feel at ease now. It's always a good idea to have an action plan for the what ifs.

I have preached so much that it is important to be in a support group. Personally I am in several support groups and I have been able to find hidden gems in each one of them. The reason it's important to involve yourself with like minded people is they understand what you are going through. Some members might be worse off than you, while others only have mild symptoms or issues. But we can learn from each other, what works best, what works worst. And in times of those meltdowns when you just need someone to listen to you or to offer you a life line so to speak. You can rest assured that several people are at the ready to come to your rescue. I can honestly say that there are times when my PTSD and anxiety is at the highest. I can count on someone in my support group to say without judgment something that makes me feel better. It doesn't always have to be words of wisdom, or someone with the right answer to make everything in the world seem alright. Sometimes just hearing someone say I hear what you are saying and your feelings are justified can be enough. I would also challenge people to actively seek out others who need to hear an encouraging word. There is no better exercise for the heart and mind than reaching out to lift others up. When you help someone else in need, the benefit is twofold. You have not only helped someone else feel better, but you also get a payday knowing you helped someone out. Even on my worst days if I can change a frown to a smile, I get a feeling of accomplishment that really changes my attitude.

Your attitude will dictate how you handle situations. I am a realist and I know that having a great attitude will not change the situation. It also won't always make my PTSD or anxiety go away. But I honestly believe that with a positive attitude, those feelings can be greatly reduced. When I look back at everything that I have been through I know that the main reasons why I am still pushing forward, why I am still here and didn't take the easy way out, is because of my strong faith in God and my positive outlook on life. I am a work in progress. I wholeheartedly want to be the person I was before my brain injury. Before I had a headache that would not go away and before PTSD and anxiety was an enemy that had overstayed its welcome. There is always hope that someday I may be that person again. But should that day never come I am ok with that. I can't be mad at where I am in my journey because of all the things I have accomplished. I have so many wonderful friends that I never would have had if my injury hadn't happened. The podcast I run with Ashley helps spread awareness to a cause that I had never given a second thought of before I became a member of that tribe. Yes there have been so many negatives that came from my injury, but there has been a light at the end of the tunnel that shines brighter every day. I found purpose for my pain.

LEAVE THE ONION PEELS BEHIND

Prior to my brain injury I had lots of things that I loved to do. I had more hobbies than I could complete in a day. I spent every morning and every evening in the gym. It was not so much of a hobby, but more like an obsession. I would work my eight-hour shift and do yard work, go for a walk, clean the house. I would tell Sheila every day: when I get off work today I am going to lay down and take a nap. She would laugh because she knew there was no chance of that ever happening. I had so much energy that I worked until it was time to go to sleep. I had no off switch and, honestly, I had no desire to find one either.

One passion of mine was cake decorating. This was something I stumbled into by pure accident. My favorite show at the time was *Cake Boss*. I just loved watching all the neat creations he came up with. On the off chance I did find down time, I would spend it watching *Cake Boss*. Sheila had learned that Buddy Valestro was coming to the Louisville palace right before Thanksgiving. She knew how much I loved watching his show and she decided that she was going to surprise me and purchased tickets for us to go see him. I was on cloud nine when she told me. I couldn't believe I was going to get to see the boss of cakes live. I didn't even mind that she was forcing me to dress up for the occasion. I still like to point out that I saw tons of people wearing street clothes. I still managed to have fun all dressed up. Plus, I got to spend the evening with my beautiful bride. That is winning any day of the week.

We got there early, and I looked around his product table and I kept coming back to his book. I really wanted to buy it, but I just couldn't justify spending that much money on myself. I've always been generous to a fault when spending money on others, but I feel guilty when I spend money on myself. Sheila saw me pick the book up and put it down several times. She finally told me to stop being cheap and just buy the book. So reluctantly I did. After I let go of my hard-earned money, we made our way to our seats. I was impressed that she had gotten such amazing seats. We were seated about four rows from the stage. They had a contest going on the display screen, if you got on twitter and sent a tweet about being at the show, he was going to do a raffle. I spent the next several minutes trying to figure out if I had a twitter account. About a minute before Buddy came on stage, I figured out how to send the first tweet I had ever sent. Of course, as luck would have it, I didn't win anything. I claim to this day that it was fixed.

The presentation was wonderful during the show. I knew how kids must feel at Disney on Ice. Towards the end of his presentation, he talked about his book, the book I purchased. He said Thanksgiving is coming up folks, I want to challenge everyone of you to go home and make this turkey cake for Thanksgiving. I looked at the photo of this cute turkey and I told Sheila that I thought I could do that. Sheila laughed her tail off and she said, "Oh you think you can do that, oh ok." Well, I have never been one to have someone tell me I couldn't do something. If you tell me, you don't think I can do something, I will do everything in my power to prove you wrong.

The next day I went to JoAnne Fabrics and purchased a bunch of cake decorating products and I was going to make that turkey cake. I was so excited to get started on it. I had the cakes already baked and cooled while I was shopping for the supplies. I bet I worked on that turkey for two hours. I followed the instructions in Buddy's book to the letter. Once it was completed, I was amazed that I had done it. Sure, you could tell his from mine in a line up. After all, he was the Cake Boss. But mine looked good. I took a picture of it and texted it to Sheila, who was still at work. A few moments later my phone rang and she asked, "Did you make that?!" I replied, "I sure did." She couldn't believe that I had done such a good job. All she could say was that it looked amazing. And so that began my little side business. She showed the cake to her coworkers and immediately they would send Sheila a picture of a cake they wanted to make and asked if she thought I could do it. It wouldn't be long before I started advertising and made my own website. I was known simply as "The Cake Baker." I had business cards made up. I was officially in business. If the head injury hadn't gotten in the way, I honestly think I could have turned this into a full-time job. My cakes were very reasonably priced and the comment I heard most often was: "This is the best cake I've ever eaten." As time went on the cake orders got more elaborate. I was blown away with each cake I made. I would stand back and proudly take a photo of my creation and was just amazed I had made that. After I had my brain injury I made one cake, and it was a nightmare. I spent over 13 hours on it. I did finish the cake, but it took everything in me to do it. The stress I endured was not worth me continuing with making cakes. I had to accept the fact that it was time to hang up the apron.

Another passion of mine was singing and playing the piano at church. As you can imagine, once you have a brain injury and have a high level of anxiety, standing in front of 200 people and singing is enough to make you feel like you are having a heart attack. So, I had to give that up and it was something that I didn't want to do. Many people have tried to encourage me to pick the microphone back up, but at this point in my life it is just something that I cannot do. As I mentioned earlier, my brain injury occurred at the start of the Covid pandemic – a time when church services were mandated to be conducted online. There was a period of three or four months that I watched from home. Returning to church was a little intimidating, the noise level of the music hurt my head even worse. I would have to wear ear plugs or go to another part of the building during the worship service. The good thing about being back in person was the chairs were spaced six feet apart in groups big enough for each family to sit together. That helped with my anxiety. I don't do well in crowded places now. I eventually returned to playing the prelude before service. That was my happy place. That was my time that I could use the gift that God had given me to give up an offering to him. Everything I played I wanted to be pleasing to God and for his glory.

After some time the six feet rule went away, and the chairs were pushed back together. The first time this happened the service was so hard for me. I felt like the walls were closing in on me. It was difficult to breathe, and I could feel my heart racing. I had to go alone that day, because Sheila had been put on mandatory overtime at work. She had to work Sunday through Friday for almost two years. It took a toll on her and she was also trying to be a caregiver to me. So that first Sunday when the chairs came back together was the last Sunday I went by myself.

It was three to four months after my prior in service church service that our current pastor had his last service before moving to Florida. I really wanted to be in person that day, I wanted to see the pastor one last time. He asked if I would play the prelude and I obliged him. Everyone loved that I played again. Everyone said they missed it, and I did too. I thought at that time, maybe I could get past the anxiety, but it was rough. I resumed going back to the online services for another month before I got brave to try it again. I got to church early to practice as I always did when I played the prelude. I walked up on stage to take my seat at the piano that morning and I saw the bass player tuning his bass guitar. I told him good morning as I was taking a seat to get ready to play what I had practiced for the last 30 minutes. He had not seen me in probably six months at that time. I was expecting him to say good morning back to me and possibly nice to see you, Rob. But I didn't get that. He sighed really loud and in such a mean tone he said, "I guess no one told you that Jim and I were going to do the prelude today." I changed Jim's name to protect his identity. I just responded with oh no, no one told me. I stood up, turned the light off above the piano, and headed back down to my seat. The bass player was still going on as I was walking. I didn't respond to what he was saying, I couldn't tell you what he said to be honest. I was mortified at the treatment I just received. I was crushed, totally devastated. I took my seat in the congregation, though I felt like I should have just kept walking out the door. I did not hear one word the new minister said that morning. The longer I thought about it, the more the tears just welled up in my eyes. I couldn't hold them back any longer. All I could do was play that moment repeatedly in my head. And the more I did, the more I cried. I managed to dry my tears by the end of the service. Normally I stick around and talk to everyone, and I am usually one of the last people to leave. I didn't do that this time. As soon as service was over, I made a beeline for the door. I made it a point to not make eye contact. I decided if I heard my name, I would keep going and act as if I had not heard someone call for me.

I haven't been back to that church since the day that happened. I totally gave up playing piano because the joy that I felt when I played was destroyed in that brief moment. It took almost two years before I would finally sit in front of my piano and play something. The joy isn't there like it was before. I've played only a few times since the day I felt so attacked. Had I blown this out of proportion? It's possible I have, but I know how I feel. Some would argue that I need to just let it go. I've spent my entire life having to hold in my emotions and conform to feeling how others think I should feel. I am proud to say I am finally at a point where I make no apologies for feeling the way I do. Will I ever find the joy in playing again? It's very possible I will, only time will tell. A few have asked me if I will ever go back to that church again. I don't have the answer to that question. There are so many people I miss. But also there are so many people that I would have expected to check in to see how I am doing, to see why I left without explanation. I am sure it's not intentional. I know life is busy and I get that. But that doesn't take the sting out of the fact that you are not being checked up on. It makes me feel like no one misses me or no one cares. Not that anyone owes me that at all, but given my circumstances and how appreciated I once was I would have thought someone would at least make the effort. I can't let the lack of compassion from others define who I am as a person. The hurt is real, but I won't let that morph me into someone who doesn't show others compassion. Please think about this with people in your life. Especially when someone makes a sudden change. You never know what they are going through. when you make the effort to check on someone you could be making a huge difference in their life – even with just a quick text or phone call.

I still mourn my old life, my old self. I look in the mirror and the man standing on the other side looks like me, but I don't recognize him anymore. I am not the same person I was before my injury. The old me would work eight hours at my job, cook super and have it ready when my wife gets home from work, do the dishes and put them away, and insist that my wife go relax. Then I would either be working on decorating cakes or be out in the yard doing yard work. I had no off switch. I would literally work from the time my feet hit the floor until it was time to go to bed.

The new me is someone that the old me probably wouldn't have been friends with. We have nothing in common. The new me gets up an hour later in the mornings now. I start work at 6AM and by 8AM I am already exhausted. I am blessed that my employer gives us what they refer to as a wellness break. We get an additional 15 minutes each day to do an activity for our wellbeing. For me that is different from the rest of my coworkers. I use my wellness break at 8AM so I can go lay down in my bedroom and be away from the computer and recharge. I can take a break every two hours throughout my workday and I use every break to recharge again so I can continue on. Some days my head hurts so bad I must use my intermittent FMLA and call it a day. But I try my best to push myself every day. As soon as I get off work my first pit stop is my bed again. I typically take at least an hour to lay down and relax and recharge. I never knew what fatigue really was until I had my brain injury.

Lately I have accepted the new me more than I did those first few years. It is hard to not miss who you used to be. Every day is a question mark. You do not know how your day is going to be until that day. That makes planning future events very challenging. You almost don't want to make plans with others because you must give them the "depending on how I am doing that day" speech. The other hard thing is the memory issues. That might be the hardest thing for me with my brain injury. I hate that post brain injury, I have a terrible time remembering. Some things stick but most do not – it depends on my fatigue and how well I am doing. If I am having a great week, I might remember six or seven days back. But my norm seems to be one to two days. There are some days that a few hours later I couldn't tell you one thing I did all day, and that is not a good feeling to have. The slap in the face that a brain injury gives you is you don't get the luxury of deciding what information sticks and what doesn't. Oh, that it could be that easy.

The plus side of having memory issues is you can watch TV shows repeatedly and it's like you are watching them for the first time. Or if you injured yourself, you probably won't remember it for a few days. I am often finding cuts or bruises on my body, and I never have a clue how or when they occurred. If you must have a memory issue, that is one plus, getting rid of the bad memories. I have told many people that I wish brain injuries could erase the bad memories from my long-term memory – the part of my brain that was not affected by the injury. I can remember all the bad things that happened to me from my early life up to the brain injury. If I could pick and choose what to get rid of, it would be those old memories. Unfortunately, brain injuries don't work that way and you have to learn to roll with punches. I can't complain about all that and dwell on what I can't have. I focus more on the blessing that I do have from my injury. I have a wonderful wife who is the best caregiver anyone could ask for. I have more friends now than I did prior to my brain injury. Friends who constantly check in on you to make sure you are doing ok. I have such a fantastic support system. I am blessed far more than I deserve.

THE GiFT OF HEALiNG

I 've done a lot of research about healing after a traumatic brain injury. There are unlimited resources, and it can be quite overwhelming. The truth is that while we all heal at different rates and there is not one specific clear-cut answer that is one size fits all. In all my research I have noticed that there are some real specifics that do check off all the boxes. One thing that all the experts do agree upon is rest. Our brain requires even more sleep once we have a brain injury. Sleep helps restore the brain by flushing out toxins that build up during waking hours. It allows the brain and body to slow down and engage in processes of recovery, promoting better physical and mental performance the next day and over the long-term. Sleep is believed to help with memory and cognitive thinking. The word I heard many times during my cognitive speech therapy was

Neuroplasticity. The theory is that sleep is necessary so the brain can grow, reorganize, restructure, and make new neural connections. I will add that consistency helps with cognitive thinking. I call this use it and improve it. Plasticity is training that drives a specific brain function and that can lead to an enhancement of that function. I read an article that summarizes this perfectly. In the article they used a technique called constraint induced movement therapy. It's used to restrain the arm on the non affected side of a patient and that forces the patient to use their affected limb as much as possible. Thereby it improved that arm's function.

I want to stress consistency as much as possible because that word is used in almost every place I have used to research the healing of the brain. Research has shown and proven that thousands and even tens of thousands of repetitions are required to generate change. I know this may seem overwhelming but think of the number of steps you take on a daily basis without even thinking about it. The more you consciously force yourself to do a task, the less it becomes a task and the more it becomes a habit. Habits are routines or rituals that are unconscious or that have become almost automatic or second nature. I became curious about habits, and I did spend more time researching than I would care to admit, but I found the following very helpful in understanding how habits help with cognitive thinking. According to Healthline.com, any habit we develop is because our brain is designed to pick up on things that reward us and punish us. When your brain recognizes a pattern, such as a connection between an action and satisfaction, it files that information away neatly in an area of the brain called the basal ganglia. This is also where we develop emotion and memories, but it's not where conscious decisions are made, that is the prefrontal cortex. This is why habits are so hard to break. They come from a brain region that's out of your conscious control. So, you are rarely aware that you are doing them, if at all.

I want to encourage you to also increase intensity. Challenge yourself to do just one thing extra than you did the last time. It really is like going to a gym. You would never get on an elliptical machine for the first time and expect that you will do an hour workout. You might start off with ten minutes and the next day push yourself to twelve minutes. The important thing is to do the work and figure out what works best for yourself.

As I've mentioned, a very important part of healing is through support groups. They are wonderful for so much more than just "support." I got a lot of great ideas to implement in my daily life just from talking to people in support groups. One thing that was so simple and should have been obvious to me was that I created a memory station. Your memory station might be different from mine, but the idea is still the same. Your memory station is one place in the house where you keep everything that you use daily. I keep my wallet, keys, and glasses in my station. Those are the essentials that you might spend hours looking for because you forgot where you laid them down. I do not allow myself to lay those items anywhere but the memory station. Since I have set this up I have never run around the house five seconds before I need to walk out the door in a panic because I can't remember where I laid them down. You may also want to keep the medication you take daily there, or as in my case my EpiPen there. That is one thing that you cannot afford the luxury of not knowing where it is when you need it.

Another way that I have helped myself to heal is by finding purpose for my life. Things really changed for me when I found my purpose. That may look different to you than it did for me. Perhaps you always dreamed of being a painter or learning how to crochet. Maybe you never tried new things because you didn't have the ambition or the drive to do so. I challenge you to find something that sounds fun or interesting to you and just do it. The worst thing that can happen is you find out that it's not your cup of tea. Then you move onto something else until you find the thing that makes you look forward to each day.

I can't stress enough how much finding my purpose has helped me. I actively seek out others who are lost and hurt so I can lift them up. It serves a dual purpose; it helps them to feel better and it gives me so much joy to know that I helped someone. That is the blessing that I keep to myself. I never feel the need to go on social media and announce all the wonderful things that I helped someone through. Those things I keep between me and the other person. Because I have been a great listener and sometimes, I have offered some good advice to others. Word seems to have gotten around, because at least once a week I will get a private message from someone I don't know that usually starts out with: "Hi Rob, you don't know me but..." I have become used to getting those now and I do my best to respond as quickly as possible. I love being someone who others feel comfortable sharing their stories with. It really is a good stress reliever to just listen to someone and help them get through whatever they are going through.

Coping strategies

There are endless strategies that one can use to help make your life easier. Some I have glossed over briefly during the writing of this book. I was able to gain great knowledge of some of these during my cognitive rehabilitation therapy. Any of the strategies that I discuss in this chapter can be altered and custom tailored to fit your personal needs.

When it comes to coping with memory issues there are lots of ways to help aid and make you feel more comfortable in dealing with the issue. The most obvious solution is to just write everything down. But I would take that one step further and suggest that you write things in more than one place. By writing something multiple times, that gives you a greater chance of remembering it. It sounds like it's a solution that is just too simple, but I assure you it is not. Writing is forcing your brain to think consciously about what you are doing. And by doing it repeatedly there is a greater chance of the important things sticking in your mind. One thing that helps me with keeping up with my appointments is not just rely on the calendar on my phone. That is super important, so you have it at the touch of your fingers, but the truth is most of us don't look at the calendar on our phones religiously. It's easy to put down that you have a doctor's appointment on June 17, but if you don't see it until June 18, then you have defeated the entire purpose of making note of it. To make this easier on me I have appointments on my phone, and I also have a dry erase monthly calendar on my wall that mirrors my phone. This way I visually see it daily and because it's there it forces me to see it several times a day as I walk by. There are zero chances of me being surprised by an appointment that I have to be at with just seconds to spare to dart out the door. The write boards come in all shapes and sizes and can be placed anywhere that you frequent most in your home. It's a very cost-effective way to keep yourself in check.

One way to help yourself not become overwhelmed with tasks is to use the timer on your phone. When you have a brain injury you lose all sense of time. It's easy to say I am going to clean this kitchen for five minutes and then find yourself an hour later knee deep in some spring cleaning. Set a realistic time that you want to spend on any given project and use the timer on your phone to keep yourself on task. Once the timer goes off you are done. Allow yourself to take a break to avoid cognitive overload and take time to rest your brain. Setting realistic goals for whatever your body and brain needs to rest will help you to not overdo it and allow yourself more energy to do other things and not stress yourself out.

Sensory overload and stress lead to fatigue, anxiety, and anger. Creating a safe space in your home that you can retreat to and decompress is an easy way to take time to calm down and relieve anxiety and anger. A safe place should be equipped with anything that you find comforting. It could be a puzzle, books, headphones, or anything that brings you joy. I will add that if you have a caregiver, get them involved in helping you set up your safe space. Discuss with them the need for you to get away to get back into a healthy frame of mind. You might be surprised to find that your caregiver may even recognize that you need to get away and decompress even before you realize it. So having them on the same page is really a great idea.

If you have anxiety when you speak to strangers in public, you may find that creating a script in advance will help you through difficult situations. When I had cognitive rehabilitation therapy, my counselor came up with a script for me based on my symptoms. She knew of my issues with numbers and she created the following script tailored just for me.

"I have a brain injury;
Please be patient with me
I want to let you know that I
Say numbers differently now
For example, I say 'ten' like 'one-zero'."

We had it printed big enough to fit in my wallet and it has been laminated. Any time I have to hold a conversation with a stranger and I know I will have to use numbers at some point, I show them my script and I have yet to have one person show me anything but support and kindness. It circles right back to education. Sometimes it doesn't have to be a life lecture to get people to understand what your needs are.

The possibilities of creating your own strategies to help you with coping are endless. And there are several apps that are available to survivors in the app store. One that I highly recommend is called in case of emergency. It's a simple app that you can use to log your emergency contacts, health conditions, medications, allergies, insurance information, as well as a section for other miscellaneous information. Once you have filled this in, all you need to do is save it as a wallpaper for your phone's lock screen. Medical staff will have this information available to them in just seconds. Here are some other apps that other survivors have suggested as helpful to them:

1. Audible
2. Cozi
3. Lumosity
4. PTSD Coach
5. Dragon dictation
6. Breath2relax
7. Mood tracker

My parting advice is that whatever you are going through, be it a brain injury, trauma, or anything in between, is that you take the time to not just get to know your (new) self, but to learn to accept yourself. You are a true miracle, and if you allow yourself to find it, your life purpose will bring you joy beyond measure. It may seem tough at this time to believe you can find your purpose, but trust me, you are worthy and a blessing.

Learning to love yourself and to give yourself permission to heal from your past traumas is a vital journey that requires patience and self-compassion. Begin by acknowledging your feelings and experiences without judgment, allowing yourself to understand the impact of past events on your present. Engage in self-reflection through journaling or meditation, which can help clarify your emotions and foster a deeper connection with yourself. Surround yourself with supportive individuals who encourage your growth and remind you of your worth. Additionally, practice self-care by prioritizing activities that bring you joy and relaxation. Establishing healthy boundaries is also essential; learn to say no to situations or people that drain your energy. As you cultivate self-love, remember that healing is a gradual process, and it is important to celebrate small victories along the way. Embrace the journey and allow yourself the grace to grow and transform.

ABOUT THE AUTHOR

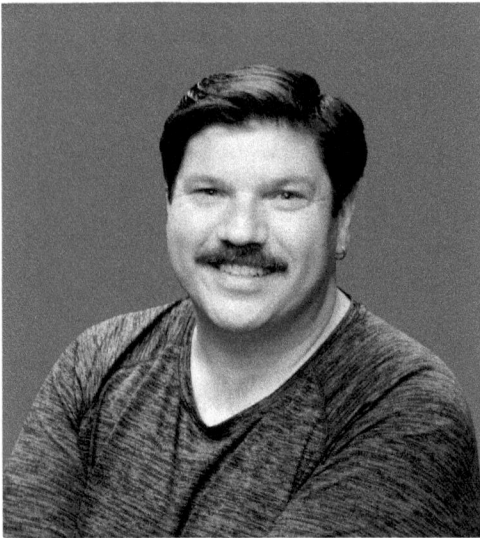

Rob was born and raised in southern Indiana. His journey with music commenced at the age of four when he began playing the piano by ear, establishing a lifelong passion that has shaped his identity. This love for music has been significant to him, yet he finds himself engaging with it less frequently due to the demands of daily life and the challenges he faces. Rob has been married to his wonderful wife Sheila for 26 years. Despite their desire to have children and efforts to adopt over several years, they ultimately chose to concentrate on cherishing their life together. Rob's competitive spirit has always driven him to tackle challenges head-on, inspired by figures like Buddy Valastro, the renowned Cake Boss, which led him to explore cake decorating at a master level with dreams of opening his own bakery. Unfortunately, a traumatic brain injury forced him to abandon that aspiration, as the high-stress environment and complexity of the craft became unmanageable. In the aftermath of his injury, Rob has spent three years seeking purpose for pain, dedicating his free time to a podcast called *Life Rewired, The brain injury podcast* that raises awareness about brain injuries, often overlooked in society. Through his podcast he talks with other brain injury survivors, caregivers, and professionals to give hope that there is life after a brain injury. Rob considers his true calling to spread joy and uplift others, while colleagues suggest he could pursue a career in comedy because of his quick wit and ability to make others laugh. He finds satisfaction in simply brightening someone's day. If Rob can bring laughter and a moment of relief to those around him, he feels that he has fulfilled his intended purpose in life.

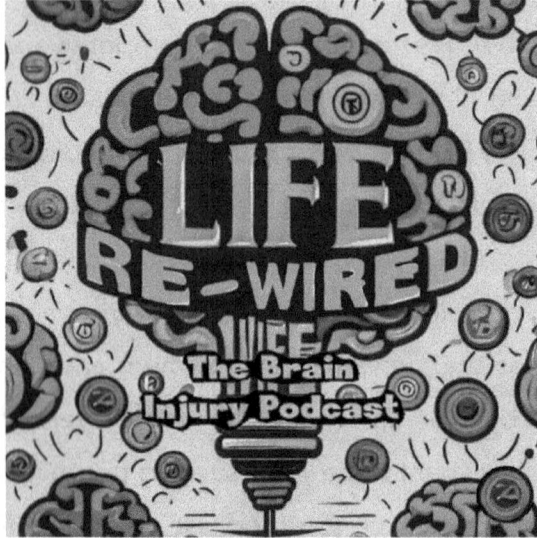

ABOUT LiFE REWiRED
THE BRAiN iNJURY PODCAST

The podcast co-hosted by Rob Baugh and Ashley Joy provides a platform for survivors to share their stories, neurotypical people to learn about brain injuries, and a support group for survivors and caregivers to show they are not alone in the world.

Like and subscribe on your favorite podcasting platform:
https://m.youtube.com/@liferewiredpodcast

ook Support Group:

w.facebook.com/groups/liferewired